MORE THAN A HEALTHY BABY

Finding Strength and Growth
After Birth Trauma

MORE THAN A HEALTHY BABY

DR ERIN BOWE

Cover design, illustrations and typeset by Elle Lynn
Author photo by Kim Selby

Cataloguing-in-Publication
entry is available from the
National Library Australia.

NATIONAL
LIBRARY
OF AUSTRALIA

ISBN 978-0-6488706-7-8 (Paperback)
ISBN 978-0-6488706-8-5 (ebook)

Dedication

For my daughters, Stella and Lily. Without their bold, dramatic entrances into this world, I simply wouldn't have written this book. You both remind me time and time again that I am strong. That if I can thrive after two difficult births, then I actually can do anything. And guess what, dear reader, my biggest hope for you is that you see this in yourself too.

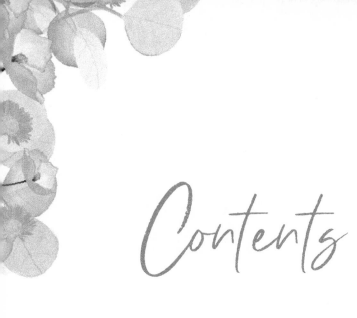

Contents

Part Two

HOW TO COPE: MIND, BODY AND SPIRIT

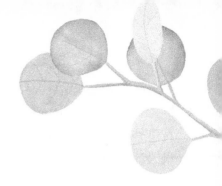

Note About Language, Gender and Bias in This Book

I fully acknowledge that I'm a white, heterosexual, overeducated cisgendered woman. Most of what I know about trauma is filtered through the lens of white Western medicine. I fully acknowledge that I have privilege and that I get to show up in places to talk about trauma where I feel safe and heard. I want to acknowledge that this may not be your experience, and I want you to feel welcome. For this reason, I choose to use the word 'they' instead of singular, gendered pronouns. I also use the term 'birthing woman' rather than 'mother' (though I do use those terms too). Please know that if you are someone who has given birth and you do not identify as a woman, my intention is not to exclude you, but to simply provide a phrase that is easily understood and translatable.

I acknowledge that the history of Western medicine has often relied on the abuse and torture of Black, Brown, Asian and Indigenous people. I acknowledge the traditional owners of the land I am on as I write, the Wurundjeri people.

There is an awful lot about trauma and birth that I don't know. My aim is to be inclusive and acknowledge that trauma is truly intersectional. I'm doing my best, and I acknowledge I'll make mistakes and get it wrong sometimes.

NOTE ABOUT REFERENCES TO BABIES

This book is written on the premise that most readers will have a living baby or babies. If your traumatic birth ended in infant loss or you don't have your baby with you for whatever reason, I'm acknowledging your pain. It's not my intention to exclude or make assumptions.

I hope this will still be a helpful book, and you are not overlooked or forgotten about. I honour the parent who has to get into a car with an empty baby capsule, or who has to go home and decide whether and when to pack up a nursery for a little soul who isn't coming home. I see you, going to your six-week check-up with no baby. I see you wanting to go to a postpartum exercise class and dreading the questions about how old your baby is. Be gentle with yourself.

NOTE ON THIS BEING A SWEARY BOOK

I never used to swear. In fact, I was regularly mocked by my friendship group at uni for being a 'good girl' who didn't swear. Then I fucking gave birth and had children! As I get older, I'm moving away from rules about what is 'ladylike' and 'professional' because I think some of these social mores are deeply rooted in patriarchy.

I won't apologise for swearing, but I will say this. There is research which demonstrates that swearing when you're in pain can help you feel less pain. When I was researching one of my podcast guests, the fabulous Mars Lord, I watched a video of her presenting at a doula conference and she gave this advice to one of her clients. Gently suggesting she not say 'shit' as she birthed her baby, but instead said 'fuck'. Why? Because 'shit' is a tense, tight word. 'Fuck' gets you to breathe more used air out, and open your mouth more. A fun fact, if you were unaware: tension in your jaw directly equates to tension in your pelvis.

You'll know by now after reading this page whether this book is for you or not!

NOTE ON THE COVER DESIGN

I am forever fortunate that I chose a publisher and design team who understood how much I *did not* want a stock image of a sad-looking woman staring out of a window. The florals on the cover were specifically chosen, and hand-illustrated, to reflect growth. A large portion of this book was written around the time of the Australian bushfire crisis in the summer of 2020. After a bushfire, certain trees and flowers regenerate and sprout new, lush foliage. Some ecosystems even thrive from fire. Australian eucalypts, banksias, Oregon daisy and the Californian fire poppy are all plants that thrive after incredible adversity.

You'll also see some gold cracks. Kintsugi is an ancient Japanese art of taking precious broken objects and mending them with gold so they are stronger and more beautiful. The cracks are also reminiscent of the stretch marks that many of us carry after growing, birthing and nourishing babies. Let this be a reminder that you are not broken. You are strong, resilient and capable.

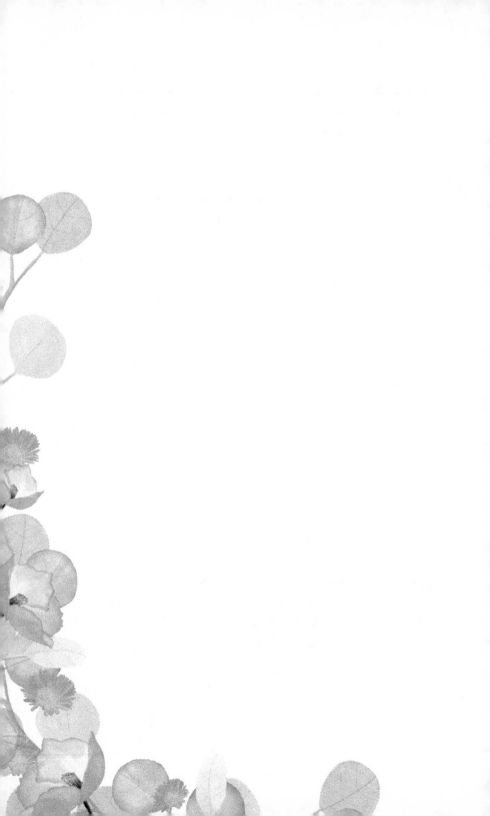

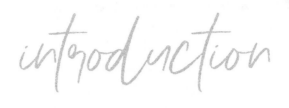

introduction

'All that matters is a healthy baby.'

How many times have you heard this and felt enraged? Forgotten about? Misunderstood?

Of course a healthy baby matters, but there is so much wrong with this statement. What about the birthing woman? Why are we being conditioned to use this reductionist language? Perhaps because there's so much going wrong for birthing women within our systems?

And what is 'healthy', exactly? A pink, chubby baby who has a loud scream and a good Apgar score? We are beginning to discover *so* much more about infant mental health that goes beyond observation. It wasn't very long ago that scientists didn't believe babies were real humans yet. They assumed that babies didn't feel pain. Now we are able to measure cortisol levels (stress hormones) in babies' saliva and understand that beneath the surface, a quiet, calm-looking baby might actually be highly distressed. The same is also true for a birthing woman. When trauma happens, people frequently have a 'freeze and appease' survival response and become quiet, agreeable and placid. This then creates inner turmoil later when they ask themselves 'Why didn't I speak up? Why didn't I fight back?'. I have much more to say about this topic.

I wanted to write a book that would make the reader feel not only validated and supported, but also encouraged. I wanted the reader to pick the book up and feel lighter, not heavier. To think this is delightfully unexpected. Trauma work is hard, but it doesn't have to be all shadow. There is lightness to be found in the work without making light of it. This is what the impact I hope to make is all about.

The focus had to be on growth. Not just a message of 'Oh, you're broken, poor you, let's fix it', but a call to arms. An authentic, heartfelt call to action for every woman who has experienced a less than ideal birth to find hope and growth. It's not even about saying we can fully prevent trauma. I honestly have come to believe that trauma is here to teach us. What is far more interesting to me is how people can find growth and strength and self-compassion despite their traumas.

I also wrote this book because, quite frankly, we're in a global health crisis and as a mother of two daughters, I simply can't sit back and just say 'oh well'. While I can build people up and be a vehicle for others' strength and growth, we also need the medical system to stop hurting people.

We have better medical care than ever before, yet attention to the needs, preferences and safety of birthing women attending hospitals is getting worse. As I write this, black women worldwide are three to four times more likely to die in childbirth than white women. In the Bronx in New York, which as I write is currently the global epicentre of covid-19, black women are 12 times more likely to die than white women.[1] They are dying primarily from issues that were completely preventable.

You're more likely to survive giving birth in the Gaza Strip than you are in Indiana.[2] Birthing women in Indiana are 11 times more likely to die than birthing women in California.[3] Data from the Indiana State Department of Health indicate that women in Iraq and the Gaza Strip have a better chance of surviving childbirth than in Indiana. Read that again.

Indiana's maternal mortality rate is 41.4 per 100,000 live births for white women and 53.4 per 100,000 live births for black women.[4] In comparison, in Australia, it's roughly 8.5 deaths per 100,000 births, with higher rates for Indigenous women.[5]

Worldwide, one pregnant woman or newborn dies every 11 seconds, mostly of preventable causes, according to UNICEF, the World Health Organization, the United Nations population division UNFPA, and the World Bank Group.[6]

If you make it out of hospital alive, then there are further systemic problems with postnatal mental health, and in particular suicide risk. Suicide is one of the leading causes of death in new mothers.[7]

Gaslighting, erasure and racism. Coercion, psychological and physical control. Maternal and infant death is just one part of the birth trauma picture. So, you see, this is about so much more than a healthy baby.

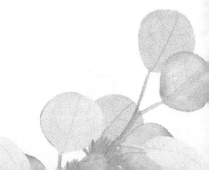

Part One

INFORMATION AND EDUCATION

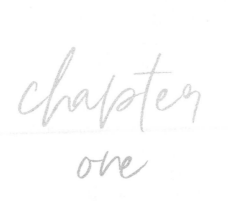

chapter one

My Birth Stories

My birth stories are beautiful, but raw. I share them so that you know where I'm coming from and what I've worked through—and that you are not alone. This is not simply a professional 'how to' book for me, this is my life. These are my births and my joys and pains.

It's hard to write a birth story that is honest and heartfelt while being mindful not to retraumatise people. I've also shared these stories on my podcast *Birth Trauma Training for Birth Workers*, and they are among the most listened-to episodes. If you're feeling vulnerable you can skip these stories or come back to them later.

> *I'm being wheeled off to emergency surgery. I'm in so much pain that death would be a welcome relief. I see my husband holding our brand-new baby girl in her little grey bunny-printed onesie in his arms and as I wave goodbye I think 'I'm never going to see you again. Please take care of her.'*

Every time I speak, write or even think about this memory of my first birth with my daughter, Stella, I well up with tears. Recovery from a traumatic birth doesn't mean that you'll necessarily ever look back on it and feel positive, or even neutral. The phrase 'get over it' needs to come out of your vocabulary right now. Instead, what I can help you with is to get through it. Not with platitudes about time healing all wounds, or focusing on gratitude for your healthy baby. Fuck that. I mean you'll go to the place where you still have big, uncomfortable feelings, but you'll be able to wade through them. Every time you're able to sit with the uncomfortable feelings, you'll get just a little bit stronger.

Surviving one traumatic birth unfortunately does not give you a free pass to avoid another one. With my second birth with my daughter Lily, I did loads more research. I had way more support, and I was more assertive about my body and my preferences. I still ended up with the arm of my obstetrician inside my birth canal rotating a five-kilogram baby with shoulders like concrete out of my body.

I didn't set out to be the poster girl for birth trauma. I would have been very happy with a peaceful, straightforward birth with fairy lights and lotus flowers. The kinds of births that so many of my hypnobirthing and birth worker colleagues have had. It's not fucking fair.

But where there is an ability there is a responsibility. I am in a privileged position. I am able to write a book on birth trauma from both the lived experience with two traumatic births, and the professional expertise of being a clinical and perinatal psychologist. I understand the research, and how to find growth after trauma.

This has allowed me to move from a place of 'it's not fair' to loving and accepting what is, and seeing that I have a message to share with the world, and if it's not me who stands up to share it, then who else is going to?

I can't ever promise to know how you're feeling right now. Trauma is subjective. People might argue with you about the details of your birth—did X and Y really happen the way you think it did? Was it really that bad? Can't you just focus on having a healthy baby? No-one can argue with you about how you feel. Your birth and how you feel about it is yours to own, so own it. Trauma is in the eye of the beholder. It's not for someone else to decide how they would feel about it and tell you to do the same.

There's also no magic cure for trauma. I think of it as being similar to weight loss. If there really was some magic formula that had every body be the same size, then we'd all be doing it, and no-one would be struggling with results, right? With that kind of reductionist thinking there's no room for individual differences, genetics, epigenetics and culture.

Working with your trauma is the most uncomfortable work you're probably ever going to do. As I write this today, it's two and a half years since my last birth. I'm still doing the work. To me, personal growth, resilience and strength mean I'm always working on something. Learning about yourself and adapting to the shit that life throws at you means you're committed to being a lifelong learner. I know this for sure though—I am strong. I can hold a lot. Physically, emotionally and spiritually. I don't have all the answers but I do have a range of tools and strategies I can teach you to make it so it doesn't hurt quite so fucking much. I trust it, because I've lived it. So now, I hold the seeds of change in my palm, like dried dandelion seeds. Let me blow them your way and see if you can let the information land, nurture it and watch it grow. Yes, something absolutely unjust, unfair and shit happened to you. Will you let it break you? Or will you find beauty from the broken parts, get back up again and find an even stronger, more resilient, more beautiful version of yourself. In spite of what happened during your birth(s)?

You didn't have to have the experience of a traumatic birth in order to grow. Post-traumatic growth is about finding positivity from a place of despair. It's about realising that if it wasn't a birth, then it would be something else and you'd be in that section of the self-help aisle. Grief, loss, illness, injury, betrayal. Same stuff, different title. It's about realising that to be human is to suffer, and learning from suffering. That you are likely to have more traumas ahead of you, because you are human.

Working through trauma is not about shifting between dichotomies. Good–bad, diseased–cured, strong–weak and so on. I hate binaries, which is why I'm a psychologist and not a lawyer. They love categories—innocent or guilty? Will the person reoffend or will they not reoffend? Psychologists annoy lawyers because we say things like 'it depends on the degree to which …'. You're not looking to get to a place of 'recovered' or (ick) 'cured'. It will depend on the day, the month, the week, the hour and even the minute. Some days will be harder than others for years to come, no matter how much time has passed. I say this with my professional hat on, because I've met people who were just as distressed by a trauma that happened 20, 30 or more than 40 years ago.

So, let's get into the stories of my pregnancies and births. I've tried to keep them succinct but I haven't censored the details as much as I have in the past. I know that reading the details of someone else's birth can sometimes trigger thoughts, feelings or memories you haven't explored before. Go gently with yourself as you read. It might be triggering for you. Stay present to what it feels like to be in your own body in the environment you are in during this moment. I'll refer to this practice a lot throughout this book. Take breaks, skim and come back to it, do what you need to do in this moment.

BIRTHING SUPERWOMAN IN 90 MINUTES: THE BIRTH OF STELLA

I wrote my birth story as a letter to my daughter, about one month postpartum.

You were due to be born on 16 November 2015. Of course, it was just a guess date and only 5 per cent of babies are actually born on their due date. Having said that, all your scan measurements were spot on, my dates were spot on and well, your daddy and I like to be punctual, so we sort of thought you would show up. I was born on my due date, but your daddy, being a twin, was born nearly three months early.

When I was in my third trimester with you, I felt pretty good. The hyperemesis gravidarum (extreme morning sickness) had left, and I really didn't feel too uncomfortable. I liked feeling you move around in my belly. When we moved to the country from the city in my third trimester, I really had to get my driver's licence. I crammed the lessons in and passed the test at 38 weeks. I kept saying that you could stay in there as long as you like—just don't come before I have passed my test! Famous last words. You did stay in there for a while, but after I was diagnosed with gestational diabetes, our obstetrician gently suggested you might need a nudge to reduce the risks. Thankfully, induction wasn't discussed until we were past 40 weeks, and we compromised and booked an induction for 41 weeks and two days, with the 'extreme unlikelihood' of needing it, according to our obstetrician. Ha!

After not sleeping much the night before, we got up at 5 a.m. to be at the hospital at 7 a.m. I was nervous. I really didn't want to be induced. I wanted labour to be as natural as possible, and knew there were risks with induction. Mostly I knew that the synthetic oxytocin could make contractions more intense and that we'd miss out on that early stage of labour. I also knew that you could get stressed at being evicted artificially and that this could increase the likelihood of a chain of other interventions. Yet, Daddy and I were both really fed up by this point. People kept asking if you'd been born yet (why do people do this?!) and we were both on high alert for any signs that you might be coming. I'd had 12 days of regular Braxton Hicks contractions, and each day that passed I was sure they would increase, but they didn't. I was dilating surely, but slowly, practising my hypnosis, sniffing clary sage until I felt woozy and doing everything reasonable in my power to convince you to make your debut. It became exhausting and disheartening. If it hadn't been for the diabetes, you probably would have arrived at a leisurely 42 weeks, but unfortunately, we didn't have the luxury of waiting. With my diabetes we needed to be careful that the placenta wasn't breaking down too much or that we were losing too much fluid.

So, on the morning of 25 November we drove to the hospital knowing we'd have a baby in the next 24 hours. It seemed like a good day to be born. The morning sky was a beautiful, rich pink and we watched as the rest of the world went about their business. I never used to be a 'pink' person, and yet after that morning I began to see the colour pink in a whole new way. Every time I'm up early (which is a lot these days!) and see a similar pink sky, I'm immediately brimming with love as I remember how much I couldn't wait to meet you. So many times, we'd driven this route to go in to the hospital for monitoring and we'd thought that 'one day' we'd be driving in and I'd be having contractions. We joked that we got to skip the nervousness of not making it to the hospital on time, and there now was really no chance of you being born in the shower or by the side of the road. When we got to the hospital, I was so excited. I strutted down that hospital corridor like I was in a Beyoncé video with a wind machine in my hair. Yet when I was greeted by that first midwife, she didn't quite share my enthusiasm. She'd just come off a night shift, so instead of throwing glitter, she simply yawned and handed me a clipboard. There were forms and lots of waiting. We met the lovely midwife who said she would be assisting with delivering you. She said that she might even get to meet you if you were born by the end of her shift—three o'clock.

At eight o'clock our obstetrician came to break my waters. I reminded her that we weren't supposed to need this scheduled induction, and she shrugged and said she was equally baffled. 'Oh well, let's have a baby now.' Her funny, casual approach was always great throughout my pregnancy. No drama. No panicking. No threats about what we weren't 'allowed' to do, and as much as possible it was a baby-centred approach to birth. She was always supportive of hypnobirthing and up to date with research. She was like the lifeguard who hangs back and allows you to enjoy the ocean, but my word, when things started looking a bit choppy (which I'll get to), she dived in calmly and helped me navigate the water.

Having my waters broken was weird. There was a lot of warm liquid. Not the kind of thing you could miss. After that, I was given a drip in my hand, and I was given saline to start with. Then at nine o'clock they started the synthetic oxytocin. I was hooked up to a portable drip and two monitors across my belly which measured the contractions and your heart rate. I got to put on some funny disposable underpants and a birth ball to bounce on. It seemed slow at first, like period pain, or practice cramps I'd had before, but it built fairly quickly after that. In hypnobirthing we learnt about using light-touch massage, having a shower and listening to music. That all went out the window, and I very quickly wanted firm pressure on my lower back and to use a heat pack. I stood up and leant over the bed into some pillows as the contractions got stronger. Having my face in the pillow helped to tune everything else out.

I would liken those strong contractions (surges) to being in the ocean with very deep, rolling waves. With the waves getting closer and closer together, I had a choice—panic, tense up and risk getting pulled under, or completely surrender, let my body flop like a rag doll and let the waves wash over me. Using surge breathing techniques really helped me to stay in the zone without feeling trapped.

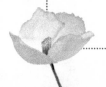

It wasn't long before the contractions got stronger and the midwife asked if I felt like I needed to push. I wasn't sure that I did really—I just felt a lot of pressure, a bit like being really constipated. I knew that meant your head was coming down and I couldn't wait for it to be out! I quietly went through transition where I thought it was going to take too long, I couldn't do it, I wanted my mum and I started to get teeth chatters. I didn't say anything at the time, and just tried to concentrate. At some point, I was asked if a student could come in to observe. At the time, I was screaming in my head 'Are you fucking kidding me?', but I said a polite 'no thank you, not today'. Birthing women are so suggestible. It's a funny place to be in, thinking that you still need to focus on being polite to people when you're in the middle of popping out a baby.

The midwife suggested I get up on the bed, because my legs had a bad case of the wobbles, and I leant into the pillows again on all fours. The surges got stronger and stronger and I tried to concentrate on imagining that each one was a big wave I was jumping over in the ocean. In between being in a deep, concentrated but relaxed state I could hear my obstetrician come back in. The nurses had apparently placed bets on when you'd be born, with the idea that there was 'no way' a first-time mum was going to give birth by lunch. We showed them. My obstetrician and the midwife were talking and I remember that it seemed really loud and almost wanted to tell them to be quiet but didn't want to break my concentration.

At some point, the funny disposable knickers came off and the deep breathing turned into bearing down and pushing. I heard myself making deep noises I barely recognised as my own voice. In fact, at one point I thought 'What is that noise? Is it a cow? No, gosh, it's me!'.

Again, I'd read about this in Ina May's book, but I hadn't grasped how *primal* birth is until I went through it myself. There was no screaming, or swearing or even moaning really, just deep vocalisations. It was hard work. In between surges I had random thoughts like thinking I should tell your daddy to remember that we parked on level four, and the words to the song 'True Colors' in my head. So strange. I bloody hate that song, and yet, ever since you were born it has popped up during interesting synchronicities in my life.

Before too long, I heard someone warning me about the 'ring of fire' when your head came out and that I needed to listen to them tell me when to push and when not to. I remember thinking that I'd decide that for myself, and got distracted by the Johnny Cash song playing in my head. At the time, I didn't realise that they were trying to prevent me from tearing since you just shot out so quickly, and, as it turns out, your little hand was in the way. I felt stinging and then relief. Phew! I felt like your head must be out—what a relief. With the next push my obstetrician wiggled you around a bit to help your shoulders and said something along the lines of 'there's a little hand'. Your hand was poking out when you were born. Daddy saw it all despite previously telling me he was going to 'stay at the top end'.

I felt enormous relief when the rest of your body slid out. I knelt up on my knees, and my obstetrician passed you through to me. We had a couple of minutes to look at each other and then we attempted the awkward task of turning over to sit upright while I held you, and the obstetrician and the nurses cleaned me up. The first thing I said was 'Oh, there's a baby!', then I said happy birthday to you and I thanked everyone for coming. I felt really relaxed, and happy and just kept looking at you. It was pretty cool. I was surprised to look and see the obstetrician stitching me up. At that stage I needed two stitches for a small external tear. My obstetrician asked if I even broke a sweat and said that I was meant to birth babies. Yes! We did it!

They gave me an injection in the leg to help to deliver the placenta (which I didn't really want but hadn't realised was necessary as part of an induction). It was OK, but the feeling of the placenta coming out was a bit weird. It looked healthy, with no signs of wear, and I remember it was a lot bigger and 'juicier' than I expected. There was no rush to cut the cord. My obstetrician actually had to remind herself that to move you over to be weighed we still had to cut the cord. It had turned from deep blue to pure white like calamari! I cut into it thinking it was just like that.

We then had a bit of time alone as a family, and I don't remember much about that. I do remember our midwife saying it was an amazing, beautiful birth and I was in the zone and that hypnobirthing obviously really works. Everyone said what an amazing job we did and when I asked how long I was in active labour I was just as surprised as everyone else. A total of 1 hour and 35 minutes for you to be born. Induction or not, our obstetrician thinks you would still have come that quickly and noted that for future, I'd be best going to hospital soon because I birth babies quickly. Funny, your grandmother was in active labour with me for only two hours and also needed stitches because I came out quickly.

Thanks to your little hand presenting in the way it did, there were some unexpected complications in the hour after birth and I really needed to focus on the affirmation of calmly meeting whatever journey birth takes. I've dealt with this part separately, but here I just wanted to focus on the birth itself, which despite intervention was great. In sum, your birth was very calm, focused and quick. I concentrated on my body and your body working together to meet a goal and when you came into the world you were very calm, alert and healthy. Without hypnobirthing I think I could easily have panicked at the intensity of it all. I can see why women are 'warned' that the contractions of synthetic induction are way stronger, but I think it's dismissive and fear-mongering to suggest that they 'won't be able to cope' without an epidural or pain meds. By knowing what was happening to my body and what it needed to do, I was able to experience 'pain' as nothing more than sensation and focus on the joy of meeting you, rather than waiting for some awful experience to be endured. I don't think I have a high pain threshold, nor am I stronger, or a better coper than anyone else. I honestly think the key to a good birth is preparation. Understanding the physiology of birth and relaxation—anyone can do it!

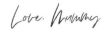

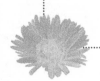

So, I really gave the *Reader's Digest* version here. I previously used my birth story as copy for my website when I was teaching hypnobirthing classes to new couples. I felt it was a fine line between sharing my story and spreading negativity and scaring people off. I had similar feelings about including too much of the negative stuff in a letter to my daughter.

The birth itself was OK. Really it was. It was fucking intense, but not painful. That's useful to know when I go on to tell you that the pain I felt about an hour after the placenta was delivered was the worst pain of my life.

It started as a dull ache. A pain in my arse. Literally. I don't know how else to describe it. When I had a midwife trying to shove a baby with low blood sugar onto my boob to get her to feed, it hurt. In addition to the bruising and blood blisters on my boobs I felt like I just couldn't get comfortable because my bum hurt. I was shifting from side to side and my midwife gave me a heat pack to lie on suggesting maybe I'd bruised my coccyx. I didn't feel right, but at this stage the general tone in the room was that a fast labour with an induction and some tearing was probably going to feel uncomfortable.

But it was more than that. I remember asking if we could try breastfeeding Stella later, as I felt really uncomfortable and just wanted to sit on the toilet for a while. I didn't need to wee, I just intuitively felt like I needed to sit on the toilet. When I got off the bed there was blood. As a first-time mum, and not medically trained, I really had no idea what a normal amount of blood was supposed to look like. I sat on the toilet and felt instant relief. Again, no wee, but an intense feeling of pressure left my body.

The details get a bit vague for me here, but I remember attempting a shower and again there was what looked like a lot of blood. I sat down on the chair in the shower as I felt like I was going to pass out. I remember being ushered into a wheelchair and being wheeled the two-metre distance back to bed. I saw an older midwife raise her eyebrows to another midwife. That was it. I knew from her expression something was wrong, and I think my body began its descent into fight-or-flight mode. Of course, once you start to panic pain starts to amplify.

Somewhere in the details here I had a catheter inserted. I kept saying I wanted to sit on the toilet, yet wasn't urinating so I guess they thought I did need to empty my bladder but was having difficulties with doing so. I remember thinking I hated birth because it just seemed like too many incidences of things being inserted in your body. Needles, IVs, fingers, hooks for breaking my water and now a catheter.

I remember being so distracted by the pain in my back/bottom area that I didn't care about anything. A paediatrician came to visit and I was thinking 'I don't give a shit. I actually don't even care about my baby right now. I'm in pain. Why am I in so much pain?'. It's funny the things you remember. I recall the paediatrician was the first one to dress Stella because I was completely distracted by pain. I recall seeing her struggle to figure out how to put the outfit on Stella, thinking that was weird for someone who worked with infants all day, and then thinking all I could do was try not to move so this pain would leave me. The paediatrician said she'd come back another time and I remember lying there waiting for what seemed like an eternity for my obstetrician to examine me, as clearly something wasn't right.

There was a shift change. A new midwife saw how much pain I was in and offered me gas and air while I waited. I think it was actually the first time I'd been offered pain relief. I had to wait for the obstetrician in order to get anything stronger. Gas and air were OK, but the effect was short-lived and made me feel woozy. I remember another midwife saying 'it's like the *Texas Chain Saw Massacre* in here'. I'm sure she was trying to be funny and keep things light, but the visual image of all that blood has never left me.

My obstetrician attempted to do a vaginal exam on me. I say attempted because the scream I let out when she attempted was enough for her to say 'OK we're going to emergency surgery'. I couldn't wait to get that general anaesthetic. I wasn't worried, I just wanted the pain to be over. The room filled with people, and an anaesthetist asked if I wanted a spinal instead. I thought 'are you fucking kidding me? I don't want to be awake for this'. He held my hand and told me I was going to be OK. He was the only person who did. When I share this part with birth worker and mental health colleagues it always attracts surprise, because anaesthetists have a reputation for often being a bit cold. Bedside manner is so important, and yet time and time again I see it gets overlooked. People forget how it feels to be the patient lying on a bed while people prod and poke and talk about you as if you aren't even there.

Being wheeled into the theatre with its bright lights and even more people, I remember feeling sad I was here again. In January of the same year, I was being wheeled in for a dilatation and curettage (D&C) after miscarrying my first pregnancy. The pain I was in now, the grief of the miscarriage, was all just so overwhelming. I don't recall much after I woke up. Other than that, I was hungry. I hadn't eaten much since five that morning except half a sandwich just after having Stella. I remember I'd ordered a cheeseburger and mud cake for dinner. When it arrived, I was told I wasn't allowed to eat it so soon after surgery and I was brought a shitty ham and cheese sandwich on white bread instead. When I think about this now, it makes me angry. I paid through the nose for that private hospital. Your first meal after having a baby should be lush and nurturing. Back then, I was naive enough to think I didn't need to pack my own food. I didn't really know anything about gut health, Ayurveda, or about how to use food and drink to nourish a postpartum body. This, of course, is why doulas are so important!

There was no sleep that night. I don't know that any parent really sleeps that first night, but when you've had a rough birth it's not just physical exhaustion. It's your brain going over and over the details, trying to put them into a story that makes sense, because our brains like stories. That night saw constant checks of my vital signs, and constant hand-expressing of colostrum from midwives to feed my hungry baby. Arguments from midwives about whether to persist with breastfeeding or use formula. Crappy night staff who couldn't get the name of my baby or any of my medications right and who kept asking me for the details. There were tears that I was still fiercely trying to hold back because I didn't want to cry in front of all those strangers. There were blood transfusions, more tests, more milking, and the dreaded task of announcing that Stella had arrived and trying to find joy when I didn't feel any. Trying to bond with a baby who, so far, wasn't eliciting much positivity from me.

I stayed in hospital for six nights, which by many standards is a long stay. My milk didn't properly start coming in until the fifth night. When it happened, I suddenly felt really unwell and thought I had the flu. This panicked me again because no-one had explained to me that this is what your milk coming in might feel like. Breastfeeding continued to be hell (which I'll explain further in Chapter 12), and I felt exhausted, angry, confused, detached, ashamed, guilty and so many other feelings.

The day we brought Stella home I was excited to introduce her to our dogs and I set about trying to cope with my feelings by creating tasks. The desire for control was strong, which I've also witnessed in many new parents. I had to set up a feeding station, a medication station, a bathing and nappy changing station. I had to sit and write a really long email to my new baby girl. I had to take a cute photo for the announcement card, and put up the Christmas tree. I had a moment where I clumsily put Stella in the stretchy baby carrier and for the first time, I felt a little bit OK. Babywearing definitely helped me to produce oxytocin and feel safe and calm in those early days. Actually, babywearing significantly helped my mental health and bonding, as Stella was, and still is, an absolutely shocking sleeper.

Despite the ordeal of my first birth, I was keen for another baby. I knew the potential for another birth to be healing, and trusted the adage of 'different day, different baby, different birth'. This takes us to the story of my second daughter, Lily.

BIRTHING A 5 KG MEATLOAF: LILY'S BIRTH

Before you were born, we were toying with whether to call you Lily or Anouk. Lily won out since (a) we figured people would mispronounce 'Anouk' all the time and (b) we knew there was a song called 'Lily'. Stella had a song with her name in it ('Stella by Starlight'), so it seemed only fair that you should have one too. So, we set about putting Lily (my one and only) by the Smashing Pumpkins on our playlist. We've since found a less creepy song called 'Way Go Lily' by Sam Amidon, but that's a story for another day.

The day before you were born, we quite literally spent the morning smashing pumpkins. I was 42 weeks plus one day pregnant, and patience gave way to extreme irritability. I watched friends putting up their photos of Christmas trees on social media, while I still had Halloween pumpkins rotting on my doorstep.

I found myself torn between wanting to wait, yet researching statistics for babies born after 42 weeks and feeling uncertain. My obstetrician said that I 'definitely wouldn't' need an induction this time, but she wanted to book one just in case. She used that exact phrase about your sister, and I ended up being induced anyway. Something I was keen to avoid this time. We'd stopped measuring at 38 weeks when scans estimated you were already 42 weeks. Having previously written an article about big babies for Essential Baby, I knew scans could be unreliable. Yet, at 1.62 m tall, I never expected to have a big baby myself!

At 42 weeks and a day I'd been in pre-labour for a week.

It kept seeming like you were close—I was 4 cm dilated and with bulging waters, but you'd only descended a little. The week before that, we went for fetal monitoring and I started feeling crampy. The midwife who was monitoring me suddenly looked at me and asked if I was in labour. 'What? I don't know, am I?' I had no idea. Next thing I knew, staff were discussing keeping me in overnight. With your sister's birth being so quick (an hour and a half), and us living an hour away, the fear was that we'd get in the car on that 30-degree afternoon in peak-hour traffic and end up giving birth on the freeway. I excitedly called Angela, our doula and photographer, and your dad started looking for a hotel. We decided a hospital room wasn't optimal for encouraging birth hormones. Room service and a bath sounded like a much better idea.

The cramps, backache and feeling of pressure continued into the night, but by morning they'd gone. I knew this was normal, and they'd probably pick back up again with a walk. Except it was already 29 degrees outside at 7 a.m. Everything about being outside in public irritated me. The smell of cigarette smoke, people's conversations and even people looking at my belly. A little old lady in the park tried to engage me in 'oh you're big! Not long now'-type small talk and it took all of my energy not to tell her where to go (not like me!). I decided I just wanted to go home.

I had spurious labour (or 'false labour' as some arseholes call it) for the past week. I could no longer leave the house without comments about how huge I was, why 'they' were 'letting' me go so long, and why I don't 'just have an induction' or 'just get a caesarean'. Night after night I went to bed with cramps and every morning I woke up and nothing happened. Cue another appointment and my obstetrician said that the spurious labour was worrying her a bit, that the constant stop–start nature of pre-labour with a bigger baby meant I might need some help. The goal was still to avoid drugs and intervention, but her suggestion was to break my waters. I kept saying to myself 'it's OK. Even Sarah Buckley (a GP who is one of my birth nerd idols), had her waters broken for two of her births! If it's OK for her, it's OK for me.'

I'd also found myself in the situation where it was now a couple of days before your big sister's birthday. My mum, who'd already stayed with us for a month, was due to fly back home after Stella's birthday. My doula, Ange, was also due to be interstate because we all thought you'd be born by now. So, at 42+2 weeks, on the morning of 22 November, we got up at five in the morning. I gazed at the pink sky, and kept saying to myself 'today is the day I meet my baby'. My obstetrician ruptured my membranes at 7.30 a.m. I had a moment of thinking 'there's no going back now', and concerned that things would move quickly and Ange was going to miss it. I was her last birth client before going on hiatus, and I think I was subconsciously holding off labour while waiting for her to get there.

While waiting for Ange, I did all the things I knew not to do. I kept looking at the clock and letting my imagination run away with me. I got angry at myself for not doing hypnobirthing 'properly', and paced around drinking litres of water and going to the toilet a lot. I started having surges where I had to brace myself against the bench. Before too long, I opened my eyes from having a bigger surge and Ange was there. Her candy pink hair and lips transported me back to the image of the pink sky, and I felt better. In her excitement (or panic) she'd gone to the wrong hospital, and barged her way into someone else's room. That's Ange. That's the doula I wanted. A presence that cannot be ignored!

Once I let go, things started to pick up, and Ange helped me through the restlessness by making decisions when I didn't know what I wanted. She put music on, gave me sips of birthing tea, massaged oils on me and got me to move around. She had me doing deep squats, swaying and getting down on a yoga mat to move you down. I clung to your daddy's shoulders, swaying, digging my face into his body and sniffing deeply to get more oxytocin flowing.

I kept doubting whether I was really in labour or not, maybe I was just pretending I was in labour because I wanted it so much? (Hello, transition!) Around 10.30, I was on all fours with the bed raised, my face buried into the pillows. I felt hot. So damn hot. And thirsty. Ange was rubbing me with a cool cloth and it was magic. It felt like she was rubbing a thick, cold body scrub into my back and I wondered how she was able to keep taking pictures with her hands covered in body scrub. I remember being truly surprised later on that it was just a wash cloth.

Second stage onset was around 12.20, and your descent felt slow, and like I needed much deeper pushes than I did with your sister. At times, I felt the different shapes of your body coming down. I remember feeling smooth and then a bump (was that your nose? chin?) At times I thought you must be crowning already because I could even feel you retracting a little. Then I felt confused when no-one said anything about seeing your head. I still felt calm, but began to doubt why there were so many deep pushes and no baby. Second time around, I was also very conscious of the fact that I couldn't hear my obstetrician's voice. I took this as a sign I wasn't 'close enough' knowing that obstetricians typically don't arrive until showtime.

By this time, I was vocalising—very loudly. It wasn't something I imagined as part of my 'gentle' birth, but just as we teach in hypnobirthing, you can't know what tools you'll necessarily use on the day. Vocalising and using the 'horse lips' technique helped me to keep my jaw relaxed and to focus on my diaphragm. It also helped to drown out sounds I didn't want to listen to. It was quite freeing, like climbing to the top of an isolated mountain and letting out all your tension with a cathartic howl.

I found myself drifting into images of strong women. Amazonians and all the primitive iconography I'd seen of birthing women from centuries ago. I felt the shadows of fierce Viking women slipping in and transferring me their energy. I've never looked to confirm any Viking ancestry, but I have these unusual folds on the insides of my eyes ('Nordic' eyes or epicanthic folds) that point to it.

There was no giving up and saying I couldn't do it. I was determined that you were going to be born without fear. I wanted you to trust that while this experience was intense, we could handle it. On the outside, I felt reassured by hearing a few times that our heart rates were in sync, and that you were quite happy. Ange and your daddy were encouraging me. Telling me to dig deep, not to fear and that I was doing a good job.

When it got tough, the sensation of two sets of hands on me, providing counterpressure and reassurance, was so comforting. I felt such a protective shield around me. Like I was protected under a solid triangle of light. The triangle is the strongest shape, and with Ange on one side, and your daddy on the other, I felt solid.

I had another strong surge, I'm certain you're crowning now and I can hear someone say you have dark hair. Before I can get too excited, my obstetrician says very matter-of-factly that I'm going to have to go on my back. Things moved very quickly and very intensely. I was aware that things were not going as they should be, but I concentrated on my breath and the goal of moving you down. There was an episiotomy, and an urgency in my obstetrician's voice. We only found out after the birth the decision-making process that went on. Apparently, I was doing very effective pushing on all fours, but you kept retracting. Pushing for longer than an hour for a second-time mum with a suspected 'big baby' is considered a risk for shoulder dystocia (stuck shoulders). Babies with shoulder dystocia who remain in second stage for more than an hour are five times more likely to have brachial plexus injury (permanent damage to nerves that connects spine, neck and arms).[8] As you were crowning, you presented with the 'turtle sign' (bulging cheeks and double chin) which is a strong indicator of shoulder dystocia. After seeing the turtle sign, birth attendants must act within five minutes to prevent hypoxia and permanent injuries to mum and baby.

Given I had already been birthing on all fours, the Gaskin manoeuvre wasn't going to cut it, so we went through five different moves to free your shoulders and get you out. Thinking about it now, I'm reminded of an HBA insurance ad from 10 or so years ago with the 'Crocodile kid' saying: 'my leg went that way and my head went that way!' All of that intensity lasted only three minutes. It felt like a lifetime. Again, I didn't allow my mind to have the word 'pain' come in. I focused on breathing (OK, howling) through it to get the outcome I wanted. The relief I felt when your body left mine was so cathartic that I didn't even notice that the cord had been cut and you'd been whisked away. It took me some time to psychologically come back into the room and I could hear myself asking why my baby wasn't on my chest. A quick resuscitation, and you were a lovely pink.

I had very few energy reserves left at this point, and delivering the placenta was uncomfortable, so I took a few breaths of gas and air. It didn't really do anything except make me faint. I had the Hollywood movie experience of hearing people's voices out of sync with what I was seeing, as everything slowed down and I passed out. Before I fainted, I could see Ange's face looking concerned and it was then that I started to realise the seriousness of what had just happened. Everyone else (including your daddy) had very deadpan looks on their faces and kept asking me if I was OK. I remember thinking that I didn't know why they were asking and needed time to think.

As soon as you were on my chest, I began to drink you in. I knew that the best way to ameliorate any stress for the both of us was to sniff you and kiss your little face. I huffed down on that new baby smell like it was a pipe of the finest opium, and it worked a treat. I was sore and absolutely exhausted, but I felt quite blissed out. I was also feeling quite smug. Despite all the talk of 'probable' diabetes, your blood sugars were absolutely fine. Just like with those pumpkins I'd assumed must be rotting, you showed no signs of being 'overcooked'. You still had vernix and plenty of lanugo, which is almost unheard of for an 'overcooker'. My placenta, like you, was huge and juicy and showed absolutely no signs of ageing. I knew my dates were spot on, so I was proud that we defied so many expectations.

Ultimately, those three minutes of unpleasantness helped me achieve a lot of the outcomes I wanted. You were absolutely unharmed. Not even so much as a bruise on you. In our case, your shoulder dystocia was quite severe, but I refuse to say that we were 'lucky'. It wasn't luck that got me the outcome I wanted. It came down to good physical and mental preparation, choosing the right care provider, and balancing our birth team.

Your birth taught me so much about finding your own personal strength. That the opposite of a gentle birth doesn't have to mean a rough one. It taught me about choosing to let go and breathe into that vulnerability to dig deep and find a raw, primal strength. Your birth was the most powerful and the least fake I've ever felt. You can't fake anything during birth! You taught me to ask for help if we need it, and to trust that others will support us through vulnerability.

Lily my Lilliputian (tiny) baby. Not exactly! You weighed exactly 5.0 kg (11 pounds, 3 ounces). Five delicious kilos of back fat and wrist rolls. I remember saying to one of the midwives who looked after us that I wanted to smear you in sweet and sour sauce and eat you! Luckily, she didn't think I was weird. To think that I lost 5 kg in the first few months of my pregnancy from hyperemesis gravidarum (excessive vomiting). In the early days of pregnancy, I was so worried about having a tiny, sickly baby.

For a few days after your birth, I felt completely energised. I kissed your little face over and over, and I was high as a kite on oxytocin. I felt I could do anything. I kept soul searching for the 'should I be traumatised?' moment. But I relied on what I know to be true about trauma. That where there is love, support and positive reframing, there's often resilience. For those women and families who do experience trauma, it just makes me all the more passionate to support them. To work hard to ensure that every birthing woman has the opportunity for a positive outcome, no matter what journey her birthing takes.

Love, Mummy

Lily is now a perfectly average sized toddler. Though when she had her 12-month check-up and she hadn't doubled her birth weight (which is the rough guideline for baby's weight development over 12 months), the maternal and child health nurse looked very confused!

My vagina was not ruined by birthing a giant meatloaf. After Stella was born, I had one tiny stretch mark and relatively flat abs again.

After Lily, it's different. I don't have incontinence, prolapse or pain, but I have what my dear friend and personal trainer, Sonia, refers to as a 'Toblerone tummy'. The technical term is diastasis recti. It means my abs got separated and are now lumpy with a gap. If I don't think about engaging my pelvic floor muscles while exercising (such as sitting up after lying down) then I can feel my organs poking out through the gap in my abs. it's very treatable in most cases, so long as you are aware and you work with someone who is an expert in postpartum exercise. It might mean surgery down the track, I don't know. I feel I barely know who my body is without pregnancy or breastfeeding, so I'm just giving it some time to lean into what that feels like right now.

I'm not at all an expert in postpartum physiology or exercise, but I don't believe that the six-week postpartum check-up is enough to know how your body is going after pregnancy and birth. Pelvic floor weakness, incontinence, injuries and diastasis recti are not necessarily a life sentence, though. A women's health physiotherapist and sessions with a personal trainer who is qualified in perinatal fitness can do wonders.

If you see an online article about someone birthing a big baby and look at the comments section, you are pretty much guaranteed to see bullshit comments rooted in patriarchy. That big babies 'ruin' your vagina. People making jokes about 'why didn't she cut the thing out?', 'it's like your favourite pub burning down', and the assumptions that the birthing woman must be 'big' herself, or have diabetes.

I also get annoyed when people say that sharing news of pushing out a big baby without drugs is 'irrelevant' or that it's somehow an offence to people who did use drugs. I've shared this on an Instagram post that went viral. The issue is not the issue. It's your perception of the issue. Celebrating a drug-free birth is not about shitting on someone who did use drugs. Celebrating the avoidance of a caesarean section does not mean I think you're weak or didn't try hard enough if you did have one. When you have trauma and unresolved negative feelings, you'll get triggered. When you're in a dark place, everything is a trigger. I get it.

After my miscarriage all I wanted to do was zone out. The morning of my D&C, a friend texted a picture of her new baby who was born the night before. I threw myself into watching *Downton Abbey* as I tried to find a show without babies and bam, there was a gut-wrenching episode about maternal death in childbirth. When World Breastfeeding Week rolled around I saw a picture of my friend in a stunning white dress, beaming as she nursed her baby. I kind of hated her in that moment. I mean I didn't really hate her, but there I was, re-engaging with my own shame about feeding my baby a bottle of formula.

Trauma causes us to see the world through a certain lens. It causes other people to potentially see us through a particular lens too— for example, the health practitioner who misdiagnoses us with postnatal depression (more on this later). Trauma is often not just wrapped up in what happened in one single event, it recurs and is complex. So, let's begin to unpack exactly what trauma is.

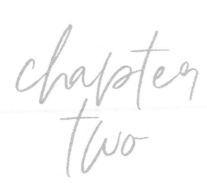

chapter two

What the Fuck Just Happened?
What Is Trauma?

I keep thinking about it over and over. I feel sick, sweaty and dizzy and my heart is pounding. I want out. I can't do this. What's happening to me? Am I dying? It's OK if I'm dying. I'm in so much pain I just want it to go away.

One in three women will experience a traumatic birth. At least this is the statistic that is usually quoted. This is, of course, a snapshot and doesn't encapsulate the broader definitions of gender identity. Nor does it capture people (and their healthcare providers) who think that they have postnatal depression (more on this later!).

Almost weekly, I'm asked by someone to explain what 'counts' as birth trauma. It's such a poorly understood term, even among healthcare providers. For this reason, I want to start by breaking it down as simply as possible.

It's with good reason that I think Melissa Bruijn and Debby Gould named their birth trauma book *How to Heal a Bad Birth*. While I'm not a big fan of categorical language, and I don't think that any birth is truly all good or all bad, it's definitely true that the descriptor 'bad' is where most people start.

Let's say you've had a birth that brought up some non-positive feelings, sensations, thoughts and memories. As the hours, weeks, months and years pass you might use different language to describe your birth experience. Here's a graduated list of terms that might be helpful:

BIRTH REGRET

Maybe you feel mostly neutral or even positive about your birth, but you experienced some disappointment, sadness, anger or regret. Let me first begin by saying that in my view, there is no 'failure' birth ever. There might be effective and ineffective choices. There may be ideal and less than ideal circumstances. Whatever turn your birthing took, please do not blame yourself or take on the idea of failure.

You might have regret about the mode of birth. For example, feeling like you wish you had opted for a caesarean instead of a physiological ('natural') birth. You might feel awkward or guilty for those choices. Personally, I have never experienced true spontaneous labour. I opted for a D&C after my first pregnancy ended in miscarriage. With my second pregnancy, I was diagnosed with gestational diabetes so I agreed to be induced after 40 weeks. With my third pregnancy, I agreed to having my waters broken (artificial rupture of membranes) after 42 weeks. Like many birthing women, I would often fantasise about what it would be like to suddenly go into labour. Would I be in Kmart and have my water break all over the floor, or would it be more like a slow trickle waking me up in the night? I would have loved to experience spontaneous labour, but it wasn't meant to be.

You might have regret about the choice of care provider. For example, feeling in retrospect that midwifery-led care would have suited your needs better than a private obstetrician. I loved my obstetrician. She supported me through a pregnancy loss and was there for the birth of both my daughters, but I sometimes wonder about the sliding doors. What if I'd chosen public hospital and midwifery-led care? What if I'd chosen home birth?

You might have regret about the birth environment. Maybe if you'd got to the hospital sooner, or maybe if you'd not bothered with the hospital at all and had your baby in the shower? Maybe you would have been fine without the epidural? Maybe you could have opted for pain relief? It's all sliding doors.

Having regret, disappointment, frustration, anger, guilt, shame or other negative emotions about birth might mean that your birth was traumatic, but it may not. A birth is traumatic if you say it is, and I still think this is the most helpful and validating concept to hang onto. But if you're finding that the feelings are not letting up, if thoughts, visions and nightmares are continuing, then this might be moving beyond 'birth regret' and into birth trauma.

LITTLE-T TRAUMA
I'm going to cover the difference between little-T and big-T trauma

later, but for now, I'll give you an overview.

You can think of little-T trauma as being a reaction to an event that doesn't quite meet the full criteria for post-traumatic stress disorder (PTSD). It has less to do with the objective details of the event itself and more to do with how you're coping with it. It doesn't mean that your birth was any less stressful than anyone else's. It means that in clinical, diagnostic terms your reactions are challenging but manageable. We sometimes refer to this as 'subclinical' PTSD (i.e. you meet a few of the symptom criteria but not enough for a diagnosis). You might also be categorised as experiencing acute stress disorder. This is like PTSD's milder form. You might have a few symptoms like difficulty thinking about the birth, avoiding thinking about it, flashbacks, panic or nightmares, but the critical point is that these experiences typically don't last longer than a month. I'll add here that I think the slightly arbitrary four-week mark was probably not decided upon by people who had newborns. What a ridiculous coincidence that around four weeks postpartum is when most mothers are experiencing acute challenges with hormone shifts, adjusting to sleep deprivation, coping with physical healing and breastfeeding challenges. I honestly think that six weeks is the minimum to even start to think about how you're coping with anything postpartum. I don't believe in pathologising, which marks the biggest change to your physical body, your relationships, your identity and your emotions. Give yourself a break!

BIG-T TRAUMA

However, let's say it's at least six weeks postpartum and you're noticing that you still feel panicked. You're having flashbacks about the birth, and you can't stop thinking about it without crying, breaking out in a cold sweat or feeling completely consumed with thoughts, memories and images of the birth. In this case, you might consider that what you're experiencing is big-T trauma, also known as PTSD. Remember that trauma is a normal reaction to an abnormal situation. Your exhausted, depleted, hormonal brain has tried to protect you from the blow of this event and now you're struggling to process it. Please know this has nothing to do with simply moving on, telling yourself not to think about it or focusing on your healthy baby. As I hope you'll learn from this book, trauma in all its forms is actually quite treatable. But it takes self-compassion, hard work and a lot of support.

Dr Sharon Dekel, a clinical psychologist at Harvard University, has recently been studying postpartum PTSD and has found that rates are between 4.6 and 6.3 per cent following full-term births. A further 18.8 per cent of women had 'clinically significant' trauma symptoms, which means a full diagnosis of PTSD wasn't met, but it was close. In 2018 there were close to four million births in the United States alone, so 200,000 birthing women in America could potentially be impacted by PTSD after birth each year. And given that globally there are close to 140 million births each year, PP-PTSD could potentially impact millions of mothers and their babies around the world.[9]

Sometimes, if you don't meet the full criteria for PTSD, what you're experiencing falls under the term 'acute stress disorder' or 'adjustment disorder'. Or maybe you have PTSD and anxiety or depression. Or maybe you don't have a diagnosis as all. This last point, that you actually don't need to have a diagnosis to have experienced a traumatic birth, is still lost on many health professionals. Each month, when I supervise other psychologists I hear stories of the policies in perinatal services. That birthing women must have an evaluation by a psychiatrist, even if they aren't even close to having a formal diagnosis. Of course, some women would benefit from the experience of a psychiatrist, but to suggest that this is the only way to receive support is ridiculous. I personally know loads of people whose response to this would be 'fuck that, I'm not seeing a shrink, I'll go home'.

The main thing for you to let sink in, and let it sink in deeply, is that trauma is subjective. Every experience is different, but with a traumatic birth most of the thoughts, feelings, memories and sensations are tied up in the birth experience.

In the *Diagnostic and Statistical Manual of Mental Disorders* (DSM-5)[10] a 'trauma' response is defined as the 'perception of actual or threatened injury or death' (to the birthing woman or her baby in this case). But see, here's the caveat to that statement. The most important factor in trauma is actually someone's subjective responses. How did the person feel? What were their thoughts, perceptions, sensations and experiences?

It's helpful to talk in terms of big-T versus little-T trauma. A little-T trauma might be that someone has what are called 'subclinical' features—they have a few symptoms like avoiding thinking about the event, anger, numbing, maybe some sleep problems, but generally speaking they don't meet the full criteria for PTSD. And these symptoms don't continue to interfere with day-to-day life after that first month or so.

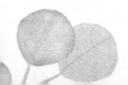

For PTSD (big-T trauma), it's different. You live in a perpetual state of panic. Even though you logically know that the event has passed, the brain stays stuck in a loop of awful feelings and sensations. The nightmares, flashbacks, the dipping in and out of feeling like you're back there and it's happening right now—that lasts for much longer than a few weeks.

Trauma is a nervous system event, not a personal failing that happened because you weren't strong enough. It doesn't discriminate, but there are some women who are more susceptible to developing trauma from birth:
- women with pregnancy complications
- women who have had a birth with interventions
- women with babies who need special care
- women who have significant injuries
- women with pre-existing mental health problems
- women who have suffered previous trauma and abuse
- women from marginalised backgrounds.

But absolutely no-one is immune from developing trauma. It affects all ages, backgrounds and education levels. Again, look at me—a PhD in psychology, a childbirth educator, a decade of helping other people with their trauma. I did hypnobirthing, I had a doula, I had an amazing birth team, I did all the research and I had a solid birth plan. I still had two traumatic births.

So again, I want to say the most important factor in trauma is subjective responses. It is *always* most important to hear and consider how the person felt. What were their thoughts, perceptions, sensations and experiences? Irrespective of what others think is objectively traumatic.

Unlike postnatal depression or anxiety (which is often misdiagnosed), a trauma response is specific to the birth and the immediate events after. Nightmares, flashbacks and avoiding thinking specifically about the birth is not a typical part of depression. Feeling panicky and anxious specifically about the birth is not a typical part of postnatal anxiety. Of course, you might feel low, anxious, hopeless, angry and numb after the birth of a baby, but again, a trauma response is a perpetual state of panic about a specific event.

I can never say this too many times. How *you* feel about your birth is what is most important, irrespective of what others think is objectively traumatic. In this way, birth trauma is in the eye of the beholder.

The same goes for people around you who may have witnessed your birth. Some partners, other family members, obstetricians, midwives, doulas, photographers (and many others) will develop what is called vicarious trauma.

When you watch something horrific happening to someone else in microscopic detail, or you hear rich descriptions of a birth story, you can start to identify with the story or even feel like it's happening to you. Sometimes, watching something happening to someone else is worse. That is not in any way to discount the experience of the person going through it, but think about this. I would take a bullet for either of my children before I would watch them be hurt. I would take all of the pain and suffering into my own body before I would watch them suffer.

Remember that the brain doesn't know the difference between what is real and what is imagined. Your brain and body will respond the same way if you simply think about something as it would if the event was actually happening. You can think about a sour lemon and have saliva pool in your mouth even though there is no lemon there. You can feel nausea and start gagging if you see someone else dry-retching, even though you have no reason to feel sick. You can think about your baby and experience milk let-down, even though your baby is at childcare. You can start yawning simply because you see someone else yawn or you keep reading the word yawn in this sentence about yawning. I have even heard of birth workers who experience 'phantom' cramping and contractions in their own uterus when their client goes into labour. An extreme case is men who experience couvade syndrome when their partners are pregnant. They gain weight, experience mood swings and backache, and sometimes even lactate. It's rare, but it happens.

Never underestimate the mind–body connection!

When you think about your own birth or witness or hear about the birth of someone else, please do not compare yourself to others and how much harder, easier, worse or better their birth seemed. If you look for it, you'll always find someone who is having a tougher time than you. In anything. Sure, using this as an anchor to bring perspective can sometimes help, but it can also minimise your own experience and thus affect your coping.

I really do believe that women in particular have been conditioned to compete with one another about birth. Instead of holding each other up, we categorise, label and organise into best/last, who had a fourth-degree tear and who 'just' had a couple of stitches. It's a way of distracting us. So long as we compete with each other the attention is taken away from those who are doing the hurting. This is an ancient war strategy: get people in a similar situation to turn on each other so that they are distracted from turning towards the source of the problem. The people in a position of power. Obstetricians and midwives who will never apologise because of their fear and ego that they might have made a poor choice. Hospitals that offer debriefs that are nothing to do with psychological support and are really just an opportunity to point the finger.

Release the need to compete with other people who've had a traumatic birth. Release the desire to look at other people (including me) and think that they seem to be coping better, more strongly or faster than you. Just as birth is so personal, our reactions to births are personal. Remind yourself that what you're often seeing is a snapshot in time. In all likelihood you're not there with someone else 24 hours a day seeing all the ebbs and flows. Often, you're not seeing them when they are in the deep of it, wading through a river of emotional diarrhoea and falling over and over again, desperate to just come up for air and feel relatively OK.

I am a huge believer in the idea that most people can hold it together for an hour. Fake a smile, put on some armour in the form of makeup or grooming, focus on another topic, or do what they need to do to convince people things are fine. Some people are experts in faking it or hiding. Maybe you already know this, because you've done it.

The same with coping. It's personal, and it's not linear. There is no trophy that's going to be handed out to whoever had the most difficult birth, or whoever coped the best. There is a wide variety of personality, developmental, cultural and social factors that influence coping and resilience.

Having a traumatic birth experience can obviously have loads of negative impacts such as:

- future decisions about whether, when and how to plan more babies
- feelings of isolation, anger, loss of control, low self-worth
- impacts on birthing and postpartum hormones—flowing on to breastfeeding, bonding, and physical and emotional recovery
- relationship issues
- trust issues
- triggering of previous trauma (e.g. abuse or assault)
- contributing to a storytelling culture that birth is bad and dangerous (which leads to more people fearing birth and higher rates of interventions).

Have you ever considered that for every negative reaction, there might also be a positive reaction? The field of post-traumatic growth is all about looking at the positive, amazing things that can happen after a traumatic event. This may seem like a strange thing to include. However, there are, in fact, a huge range of possible positive outcomes from a traumatic birth. This is not about rushing in and going 'Oh but you've got a healthy baby, you're not dead'. Not at all. I stress, these are just possibilities for when you're ready to explore them (keeping in mind though that you may never be ready).

Possible positive outcomes from a traumatic birth include:

- resilience
- improved coping
- feeling closer to your partner
- increased confidence and self-admiration
- a sense of power, bravery and accomplishment
- a big middle finger at the system (refusing to be a victim)
- having previous anxieties and difficulties fade into the background (e.g. dealing with difficulties at work suddenly seems trivial)
- the desire to share this with others and improve birth outcomes
- improved storytelling culture
- awe, admiration and inspiration.

Again, you get to find the positives yourself at some undetermined time. Finding positives after the trauma is personal. It must be one of self-discovery (the best kind of learning), with time, support and space to heal.

Maybe you've found that even very early after the birth, you've been given advice about how you should feel from people not qualified to tell you (hint: that's everyone who isn't you).

Jumping to a positive outcome prematurely is dismissive and placating, and rarely helpful. Perhaps you've had the experience of hearing: 'at least you've got a healthy baby'. Words and phrases like 'at least', 'but' and 'just' are all ways of dismissing your experience.

This might be a good place for me to share with you some of the bizarre reactions my husband and I received when we first told people I'd miscarried our baby. I was pregnant at Christmas, and as a woman in her 30s who'd been married for 10 years, I knew that avoiding alcohol, soft cheeses and seafood was going to invite comments. So we decided to tell people when I was about seven weeks pregnant. I'd always said that if I miscarried I didn't want it to be a secret. Yet when it happened the first thing I said was 'I wish I hadn't told people'. I regularly change my mind about that decision even now, partly because I got comments like:

> 'At least it wasn't too far along.'
> 'You'll just have to try harder next time.'
> 'It wasn't meant to be.'
> 'It's better than having a baby with something wrong with it.'

I'm also a big believer in the fact that when people don't know what to say, they sometimes say the absolute wrong thing. Pregnancy loss and birth seem to attract some of the worst comments, and again, I think some of this goes back to our cultural conditioning about dichotomies. We sometimes assume that pregnancy and birth are always happy, positive times. We forget that self-aware humans are capable of holding two conflicting views or emotions at the same time. For example, you can feel white-hot seething rage at your partner in a moment of sleep deprivation and miscommunication, but still love them. You can know all the risks and negative impacts of smoking, but still choose to smoke. It's called cognitive dissonance.

You can have a crappy birth and still love your baby. You can feel neutral, indifferent, fearful, resentful and angry about pregnancy, yet still love your child. You can feel angry, hard-done-by or even victimised when finding out your child has an injury, illness, disorder or other special needs. When I first found out that my first daughter had a very rare genetic disorder I was devastated. I was also pissed off, and that's not easy to admit. I'd paid for expensive genetic screening in my pregnancy, yet she has a disorder so rare, and one that's probably a new mutation rather than inherited, that there's no way screening could have picked it up. If screening had picked it up, I wouldn't have changed anything. I love my daughter, but I don't always love her condition. I don't always feel that it's great to be unique and different. I don't always feel confident that she will grow into her unique look and stand proud to celebrate her difference. When she is bawling her eyes out because she doesn't look like other three-year-old girls and is too young to fully understand why, I don't love her condition.

Stella has ectodermal dysplasia.[11] To put it in a nutshell, an embryo has three layers. One of those layers is the ectodermal layer which is responsible for skin, hair, teeth, sweat glands, tears and other related things. In ectodermal dysplasia there are abnormalities which develop in that layer, leading to a bunch of issues with skin, hair, nails, teeth and so on. About seven per 20,000 people have ectodermal dysplasia. There are at least 180 different types, plus more that have yet to be been identified. Stella's type (which we don't have a name for) can't be traced through our family history and her sister doesn't have it, so it's probably a brand-new mutation. She's like Wolverine. Actually, less like a wolf and more like a vampire. The way that ectodermal dysplasia presents for Stella is pointy vampire-like teeth and very pale almost translucent skin. Hair that is almost colourless (like a polar bear's), very fine, sparse and slow growing. She also has a few scooped nails which grow very slowly and break off easily.

As far as I know today, the way that ectodermal dysplasia affects her is mostly cosmetic. It's also emotional in the sense that we live in a world obsessed about femininity being associated with long hair. Do you know any Disney princesses with super, super short hair? There are TV shows and toys and books completely dedicated to long hair and styling that are marketed at very young children. It's near impossible to shield your child from it. And, as much I was the mum who said my children would all be in gender-neutral clothing and play with gender-neutral toys, they fucking love pink and dolls. I tried.

We deal with stares and comments from strangers thinking she's a boy. I've had grown adults tell me I shouldn't dress her in blue because people will think she's a boy. We get people thinking she has albinism or cancer. I see people treat her like she's made of glass because they assume she is sick and I can't always be bothered having the conversation with every new person we meet.

I'm telling you this, because I really, truly get what it is to deal with mixed feelings about birth and your babies. I too have swung from 'I'm so lucky my baby isn't sick' through to feeling grief-stricken that she has to deal with the burden of being different. You can hold those feelings and still know that there is nothing you would change about who your child is.

The first thing people will say upon hearing a pregnancy announcement is often 'congratulations'. There's nothing wrong with this, if this is the response that the birthing woman or couple want to hear, but already it's loaded with expectation about how to feel. I have birth worker friends, who therefore don't use the word 'congratulations' in their first conversation with a client, but instead ask 'How do you feel?'.

After congratulating you, people tend to ask if you're excited. They forget that maintaining any emotional state is not linear. You simply can't be excited all the time. Yet, I will still never forget the looks on people's faces when I answered this question honestly 'no'. No, I've just vomited for the 20th time today. I've been on a drip, I'm nauseous all the time and I still have to deal with dirty nappies and toddler tantrums, so no, I'm not excited right now.

We must stop rushing to find the silver lining in birth. No-one says 'at least you've got a healthy husband' if your wedding doesn't go as planned. If your drunk uncle falls into the cake, a toddler vomits on your dress or your flowers aren't what you ordered. People expect this to be a happy day, so they acknowledge that of course you should feel outraged if it's not right. Yet with birth, people rush to grab their proverbial pom-poms and insist on telling you how you should feel and what you should focus on.

If you have never done so, I urge you to consider the following questions:

1. What are your own early memories of learning what birth is and what it's about?
2. What were the emotions, language etc. around depictions or descriptions of it?
3. Do you have memories of specific TV shows or movies depicting birth that you watched when you were young?
4. When did your views about birth change?

Trauma, like many psychological issues, is invisible. We have the technology to scan the brain, look inside and 'see' trauma, but the majority of people are never going to get a brain scan. Diagnosis is through observation and communication. We can't cut your brain open, go 'look, all the trauma is gone!', stitch you back up and say you're cured. The medical model of 'find the problem, treat it and cure it' doesn't fit with trauma.

Many people who struggle with depression, anxiety and trauma experience disbelief and suspicion from other people. How hard is it to maintain the look of someone who is struggling with an invisible illness? Just to be believed. Human experiences are not linear, yet so many people with depression struggle to find a way through the illness because they live in fear that they are making it all up. They fear that if they dare laugh, smile or temporarily find some joy, then people (a) won't believe they are really unwell, and (b) will jump to the conclusion that they must be better.

You can enjoy your baby, giggle and have fun and still be traumatised. You don't have to keep an act up or wear a certain mask in order to gain understanding of how difficult things are for you. A huge part of my mission and message in this work is to teach that trauma doesn't have to be all dark and shadow. We can find joy, strength, humour and light, frothy fun if we want to. We can make dark, sick jokes about our own suffering if we want to.

Comedian and director Rob Reiner once said 'The Holocaust itself is not funny, there's nothing funny about it. But survival and what it takes to survive—there can be humour in that.'

Filmmaker Mel Brooks also caused quite a stir when he would joke about Nazis. He said 'Anything I could do to deflate Germans, anything, I did'.

Some people can't tolerate it when comedians make jokes about the Holocaust, and that's OK. If finding laughter in your suffering helps you, then do it. There is truly something to offend someone in every comment or behaviour we make.

Experiencing joy doesn't mean you don't have trauma. In fact, I would say that we really don't know just from looking at someone how much trauma they have. Or whether they are currently experiencing trauma when you talk to them. Sure, there are subtle and not so subtle cues, but it's not an exact science. Someone who is mid-flashback, in active trauma time, might look neutral. Even for a trained expert, it's difficult to tell if someone is stuck in trauma time. This is often why I'm wary about trauma groups. Something that someone says or does can easily be a trigger for someone else. Since you can't always tell that someone is having a trauma response (e.g. their heart could be racing, they could be dissociating but they otherwise look fine), it may go unnoticed. That can trigger feelings of being invalidated and unable to escape. There is a huge onus on the individual to put their hand up and say 'hey, I don't want to hear this', walk out or do something else to self-manage their response. Can you see then how this cements all the pre-existing feelings of being trapped, disrespected and like it's your fault?

When there is a crisis, bringing all the people involved together to talk about it can result in what's called emotional contagion. I've seen it happen time and time again in schools when my area of expertise was self-harm. Let's say there's been an incident of self-harm. The staff at the school jump to conclusions and assume the intent was suicide. Next thing you know, all these kids are brought into a group to talk about suicide. Emotions are heightened, competitiveness maybe starts to creep in, and before too long you've got a crisis on your hands. Kids who were otherwise doing OK that day are now suddenly triggered. Some of them maybe learn this is a way to get out of class, or to have someone respond to them in the way that they want. This is called operant conditioning. An example is carrying out a behaviour (like cutting yourself) that has nothing to do with ending your life, but with changing your situation or how people are responding to you.

It also happens online in groups where people who have experienced a trauma or an illness start to engage in what's called groupthink. Overidentifying with other people's symptoms and stories, becoming competitive and confusing venting with sharing. Making it into an 'us and them' situation.

Despite our conditioning through movies and TV, PTSD is not always expressed as a war veteran cowering after hearing a car backfire because it's triggered 'shell shock'. You could be sitting on a bus next to someone having an active panic attack and no-one would know.

What is your first memory of learning about 'trauma'?

My first exposure to learning about trauma as a concept was watching the movie *The Client* with Brad Renfro and Susan Sarandon. I was home sick from school, back when you could catch a midday movie that was totally inappropriate for children (hello, 1990s).

I recently re-watched this as an adult and just had to shake my head. The synopsis in brief is that an 11-year-old boy, Ricky, and his little brother are smoking in the woods near their house when they encounter a mob lawyer. This adult tells the boys he's going to commit suicide to avoid being murdered, and the boys witness the suicide. Ricky becomes catatonic and is rushed to hospital in an ambulance. PTSD is diagnosed by a medical doctor in a white coat less than 24 hours after the event (incorrect). Ricky remains non-verbal and sucks his thumb. Then this phrase is uttered: 'The doctor wants to start you on Valium'.

I know it's an old movie, but I wonder how dramatic portrayals of trauma assessment and treatment impact on the subconscious. As if there's a certain way you're supposed to behave if you have trauma.

The takeaway is that there are really no rules. There are symptoms and possible diagnoses, but there are no hard and fast rules about how you should feel or behave. Trauma is where there is too much, too fast and too soon for the body and brain to process. You feel overwhelmingly uncomfortable thinking about your birth and keep thinking about it when you don't want to. Your body reacts with sensations like you're right back there and it's happening again. Let's dive a bit deeper into why it happens. Let's look at why your body has had this response and why there's nothing you could have done, said or thought that would necessarily change things.

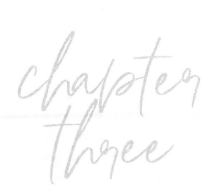

Why It's Not Your Fault:
Trauma and the Nervous System

What I'm about to explain here is something I really want you to be open to receiving. To not just brush it off, but give it a pause and let it land in your body. I want you to really take a few deep breaths here. Breathe in through your nose, hold it at the top, and then let it go slowly. Centre yourself, and be open to receiving what I'm about to say.

It's not your fault. I mean it. Let that sink in. This is not some bullshit flowery placating response. This is truth. It is fundamental to your moving forward that you can at least begin to entertain the idea that this is truth.

Your trauma did not happen because of something you did or didn't do. It didn't happen because you are weak, aren't built properly, are damaged, or because you didn't deal with your childhood stuff as well as you thought you did. Being a nurse, a counsellor, a midwife, a doctor, or having worked through previous traumas does not protect you from having a traumatic response to your birth.

It most certainly didn't happen because you aren't grateful enough. Gratitude and trauma really have very little to do with each other. Yet, with birth they are spoken about as if they are antonyms. You will not go into a thesaurus and see 'gratitude' as being the opposite of trauma and vice versa. Gratitude is also not an antidote to trauma. It might temporarily make you feel something other than traumatised, but here's a thought: you can be grateful *and* still have trauma. You can be an optimistic person, have had a great night's sleep, be in a good mood that day, and still develop trauma. You can have done all the research, had a solid birth plan, completed independent childbirth education, hired a doula, kept up with your Kegel exercises, practised your affirmations and *still* experience trauma.

Some of you at this point are going to want hard evidence rather than reassurance. I get that, so let's go into the science. Trauma is a nervous system event that happens when you are flooded with sensory information that's too much, too fast and too soon. Developing trauma means that your nervous system has worked hard to protect you from an onslaught of sensory information. Trauma is a normal response to an abnormal situation.

During trauma, we also know that the brain tends to get 'stuck' in the past. The experience of a threat makes different parts of the brain light up and some parts dull down. Parts of the brain that usually connect with each other can become fragmented.[12] If we look at trauma and the brain from a sensory processing angle, then we know that people experience things like finding it very difficult to stay in the present moment. People who have experienced trauma frequently find themselves stuck in 'trauma time', where even though a part of them may know that they're sitting in their living room reading a book, their brain is taking them back to the moment of giving birth. Knowing exactly how you feel and how to articulate it can be difficult. Being able to see into the future and figure out what is relevant information and what's not can be difficult. Having a sense of an embodied self (how you feel in your body in your environment) can also be disrupted. In complex trauma, we sometimes also see a disrupted sense of self. For example, people who have experienced long-term abuse and neglect as children sometimes don't even use the word 'I' because they struggle to have a sense of themselves as an individual with a body existing in the world.

Knowing in your rational mind that the threat has passed and can't hurt you anymore is one thing. Having a deep-felt sense throughout your whole body that you are safe is completely different. I know for some of you the desire to work through this with logic is strong. I know you've probably had countless shower fantasies about what you could or should have done or said. Maybe you've had the delightful (insert sarcastic tone) experience of being told 'it's over, there's nothing you can do, move on with your life'. Maybe it's even come from people who love you and want the best for you, but who are not experts in how to help you. Think about how many psychologists, psychiatrists, counsellors and coaches would be out of work if it were true that all you have to do is 'move on', be logical or stop thinking about it.

Trauma doesn't reside in the same place as insight. You can't 'insight' your way out of trauma. Your brain is attached to your body and your central nervous system. Going over and over and over the event by venting and ruminating doesn't have long-term effects. That's not to say that talk therapy doesn't work or isn't useful. Exploring, labelling and reframing your story with a skilled person can have life-changing results. This is why I fucking hate all the 'who needs therapy when I have you guys?' memes with Carrie from *Sex and the City*. Let us not forget the wisdom that Samantha gives in response 'we're just as fucked up as you are. It's like the blind leading the blind'. Listening and empathising is great. Here is the thing, though. There's a reason why it's unethical for psychologists to provide therapy to someone close to them. A huge part of that is because when we actually love someone, we interject and interrupt their trauma processing with all of our facial expressions. All of our normal, human responses like 'I'm so sorry that happened' and 'are you OK?' interrupt the trauma process. You need someone with some distance so that you can say what you need to say and react how you need to react without worrying about the other person's energy. For professionals, there's a knack to being warm enough yet distant enough that their presence doesn't actually impede someone else's healing. Your friends and family love you, so they also tend to refrain from telling you what you need to hear. And sometimes they are part of your trauma story and so you can't actually rely on the genuineness and consistency of their behaviour towards you.

So again, you can't just use logic to work your way through trauma. Think about the concept of an invisible illness. Think about how many people struggle with what they know or think versus what they feel. I can 'know' that my experience of childbirth is in the past, but that doesn't translate to me feeling OK about it. Knowing is not enough. Your body feels reminders of the trauma as if they were happening right now.

Let's look at how you can start to shift some of those negative feelings, sensations and memories by beginning to learn about emotions and coping.

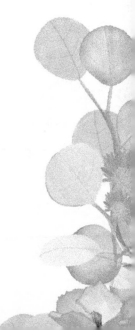

Part Two

HOW TO COPE:
MIND, BODY AND SPIRIT

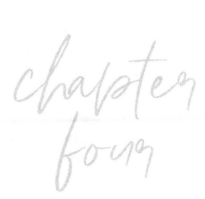

Coping With Thoughts and Emotions

'I'm not coping.'

It's probably the most popular response I've received to that first question in a session with a client, 'What can I help you with today?'

First of all, the optimist in me who gets very excited about positive psychology and growth would point out that in actual fact you are. I want you to know that picking up a book and having a go at working on yourself, that's huge. Do you know how many people are forever immobilised by their trauma and never work on it?

Making that first appointment with a psychologist or counsellor is a huge effort. I often say to clients in these early days that the fact that you got your bum on the seat *is* coping. It might not represent the level of coping you'd like, but if you're doing *something* then you can't say with 100 per cent accuracy that you're not coping.

Even if you are finding yourself engaging in maladaptive coping strategies (e.g. things that maybe temporarily make you feel good but are not enhancing your life), that's still coping. In my early career I worked with people who typically coped by engaging in all sorts of impulsive and dangerous behaviours—self-harm, risky sex, alcohol and drug abuse, violence and so on. Every single one of these people had trauma of some sort. An attempt to cope (no matter how maladaptive) is still an attempt.

We are conditioned to avoid suffering because it's unpleasant, and unpleasant things are intolerable. Our conditioning that unpleasant emotions are to be avoided begins early. We say things like 'don't cry' and 'you're OK' to small children. We distract them with food and toys and novelty so that they don't have to feel their negative feelings.

We go to great lengths to avoid unpleasant feelings, and yet I personally really resonate with the idea that this is exactly what we are put on this earth to do. To suffer and find lessons and growth in the suffering, not to keep living a life where we avoid it. Where would we be, spiritually, personally and professionally if we were instead taught that suffering is tolerable? That it's a practice.

WHAT IS 'COPING' EXACTLY?

Coping is defined very broadly as the effort or attempt someone makes to reduce the distress that's associated with negative life experiences. This is why I say that any attempt is still an attempt.

Some people categorise coping behaviours as 'approach coping', or 'avoidant oping'. You could also call them adaptive or maladaptive coping strategies. One example of a questionnaire that's used to measure coping is the brief COPE (Coping Orientation to Problems Experienced) inventory. Clinicians use it to identify the different ways that people try to cope: self-distraction, active coping, denial, substance use, use of emotional support, use of instrumental support, behavioural disengagement, venting, positive reframing, planning, humour, acceptance, religion and self-blame.

Looking at this list, you might already have some ideas about which types of behaviours you typically engage in. Knowing what are your go-to strategies, how they compare with those of your partner and family members or friends, and which ones you want to boost or reduce, can be helpful. Coping is a teachable skill, and most of us were not taught a whole lot about it by school or our parents.

If you want some practical coping strategies, you can check out my book *Practical Coping Strategies for Coping with Birth Trauma*.

EMOTIONS AND THE BODY

Emotions, the brain and the body are not separate units. If you were to draw these concepts for a child, what would you draw? An outline of a body, a lumpy shape in the centre of the head and maybe a heart shape where the heart goes? It would be a good start, but it needs loads of connecting lines. You might feel your heart pounding. Your jaw may clench with anger. You could describe the feeling of butterflies in your tummy. Most children communicate their emotions with physical descriptions saying that they 'feel sick'. Some cultures also refrain from talking about unpleasant emotions due to taboos about mental illness and instead describe 'nerves' or 'headaches'. Plenty of people go to their family doctor because they need to pee all the time, have headaches, experience diarrhoea and cramps and can't sleep. Sometimes these people are genuinely surprised when they are sent off to see a psychologist and find out that they have anxiety. You can get so used to having anxiety that you actually don't remember what it's like to feel calm or neutral. Then there are the people who rush off to the emergency room thinking they are having a heart attack only to be perplexed and often sceptical when it's found they had a panic attack, or drank too much coffee or energy drinks.

Most of us were not taught a great deal about emotions, coping and the mind–body connection when we were growing up. Instead of acquiring these skills in school we spent our time learning other useless bullshit (please read that tongue in cheek, I wouldn't have spent 24 years in formal education if I really didn't value it!). But seriously, at my high school we even had a class called 'life skills'. And to use another 1990s quote from the movie *Sister Act*, you could call it a 'bird course' because we flew right through it. As far as I can recall, public schools in my area were left with a miscellaneous section in the timetable because we weren't doing religious studies. Other than the occasional lesson on how to write a job application and why you'll never get a job if you have long hair (if you're male), or have piercings, dyed hair or tattoos, we didn't do much. In fact, much to my loathing, my home-room teacher for two years in a row was a physical education teacher, so it meant we 'got to' spend these lessons playing cricket. Well, most of the class did that. My friends and I swapped Tazos and debated which Hanson brother was hotter. The point is, I look back as an adult and see such missed opportunity for the teaching of actual life skills.

You would have heard the expression 'it's all in your head', a dismissive statement used to mean all sorts of loaded things. The thing is, it's true! It is all in your head, and you know what? Your head (brain) controls every single part of your body, so how can it not be in your head?

Talking about it might not be enough. Bessel van der Kolk says that if people can talk about it (the event) then it's not the most traumatic part. My personal view is that most people benefit from a holistic approach, something that incorporates both body and mind as an orchestra playing together, not as separate isolated tracks.

THE AIM METHOD

As a starting point, there's an acronym I've come up with to help remind you what to do to cope after a traumatic birth. It sums up what I think is important to integrate mind and body after any event that's left you feeling rattled with images and memories that are intrusive.

A for Allowing

I for Integrating

M for Meaning Making

Step 1 is allowing. Allow whatever you feel, whatever thoughts you have to just come in. Without trying to push them away or distract yourself. Telling yourself not to think about something won't work. Again, think back to what I said earlier about how mental health professionals are able to keep employment. The simple fact is that telling yourself not to think about something actually doesn't work. If it was as simple as 'just don't think about it', I wouldn't have a job. I also wouldn't have wasted my time getting that PhD.

The technical term for 'why just don't think about it is bullshit' is ironic process theory. The more you tell yourself not to think about something, like a pink elephant, the more your brain will keep firing information about pink elephants.

Try it. Don't think about a pink elephant. You can think about whatever you want but don't think about a pink elephant. You're not allowed to think about it. Don't think about it. Just stop thinking about it and think about something else. How did you do?

Instead, what you're aiming to do is the opposite. Allow the thoughts that you don't want in for small doses—twenty seconds at first, then two minutes, whatever you can do. When you train your brain to allow this it will help reduce future fire-ups. Allowing is not the same as liking. You don't have to like the thoughts and feelings, just let them in.

Step 2 is integrating the story. Your brain wants a story with a beginning, a middle and an end. Your brain is like a giant filing cabinet. You need to tell it where to organise things so that everything doesn't spill out. You don't need to go back and remember every detail. You don't need to interview everyone who was at your child's birth at get their take on things. There's a reason why police will often try to separate witnesses to a crime or disaster. When people get together after a traumatic event and swap details, they become highly susceptible to influence from other people. Focus on how *you* feel in your body and what *you* think happened. To this day, my doula, Angel, will say 'Oh, this happened at Lily's birth' and I'll have no recollection of what she's talking about, or I'll remember things differently. That's OK. You are the main player here. All you really need is a simple story for what happened, retold to yourself in a way that feels OK for you. Remember, accepting is not the same as liking. You don't have to let it go or make peace with it yet, just allow the story to be what it is.

Step 3, the final step, is meaning making. What are you going to make this experience mean? That you're a failure? That you're weak, that you should feel guilt and shame or that you are strong? That if you can get through this you can get through anything? Find the growth. What could you learn about yourself from this? What did you do well? Change the story. I'll say it again. This is *your* story. You can make it a Greek tragedy, or a comedy or a dramedy.

> **If you get stuck, think of an 'if then' statement:**
> 'If I birthed a five-kilo baby with severe shoulder dystocia, then it means I'm strong as hell.'
> 'If I've made it this far, then I have a hundred per cent success rate at surviving.'
> 'If I survived the trauma, then I can survive the work to heal it.'

Once you've got your story, you are likely going to have some big, uncomfortable emotions and weird bodily sensations. Let's look at ways to quickly calm your nervous system.

SIX SENSES SELF-CARE STRATEGIES

Think of these like a HIIT (high intensity interval training) workout for your brain and your nervous system. These are macro or general strategies. This is not the deep dive work; this is the paddling around in the shallow end to warm your body up. This is a bunch of my go-to strategies for when you simply need to change and shift your emotional state.

Recognition is far easier than recall. If you have a list on your phone of things to do when you feel stressed, this will be much easier than waiting until you are an emotional wreck trying to come up with something to soothe yourself.

Let's start with engaging your visual senses.

VISUAL

Use a grounding image on the lock screen of your phone. Don't go people-pleasing. I know your kids are cute, but at the moment this is not about them, it's about you. So, what's something that really lights up the pleasure centre of your brain? What's an image that reminds you to check in with yourself and why you are doing this? Mine at the moment is a picture of me at the age of two or three. At the time of writing this book I've been doing a lot of inner child work with a coach. Like many nurturing healer/helper types I have a history of giving loads of my time and compassion to caring for others, but giving none to myself. Seeing little me reminds me to take care of myself.

Do you have a folder or a playlist of videos that light you up? What gets your endorphins flowing? There is real research[13] behind the benefits of watching funny animal videos, so I'm all for that.

Healing is not all serious and dark. Finding joy in meaningless, silly or childish videos can be part of finding the fun again. So, do yourself a favour and go watch Sophie the bulldog roll down a hill—that's one of my favourites.

If you have tattoos and they are meaningful to you, do you actually spend the time to look at them and check in with their beauty and meaning? Or have they become second nature and you don't give them a second glance? Revisit the purpose and intention behind them. Trace your own skin and get some oxytocin flowing. If they are no longer positive, then seriously make a plan to get them changed or removed.

If you are not a tattoo person, could you find some temporary tattoos or draw on yourself with positive affirmations? When I've worked with people who engage in self-harm, one of the ways of shifting through replacement coping skills can simply be writing or drawing on themselves. Did you ever write on your thighs under your school dress? It might not have been particularly meaningful (EB 4 JB 4 EVA type stuff), but go back to the feeling. The intention, whether you knew it or not, was to get a dopamine hit. A little shot of happy, natural hormones. Did it feel exciting or forbidden? What would happen if you got caught? Would you get suspended, expelled from school? Can you actually die of ink poisoning from writing on yourself with a biro? (No, Mum, you can't.)

If you're not into that, then it might be practising closing your eyes and seeing a snapshot image in your mind. You in your happy place—on holiday or maybe in a totally made-up place. Fantasies are free, so where do you want to go? A lush rainforest surrounded by wild, powerful yet totally tameable animals? That's one of my happy places. What did you daydream about at school?

KINAESTHETIC

Kinaesthetic strategies like using 'horse lips', blowing raspberries and using yoga or tai chi movements help release tension. They keep our own oxytocin and serotonin flowing. For women in particular, tension in the face equates to tension in the pelvis. If you've ever come across Ina May's work in birth, you'll know that she talks about the importance of an open mouth and relaxed jaw for birthing.

Letting go—both letting go of tension and letting yourself become free—means laughing without controlling or tightening your face. If you laugh like a hyena or snort, so be it. Give yourself permission to be your unhinged self. Let that jaw go. Laugh, sing, cry, scream and orgasm with your mouth open.

Mindfully wash your hands. Massage your hands, and bring awareness back to your body. You know that phrase 'I know it like the back of my hand'? Do you actually know the back of your hand? Look at it, describe it to yourself. Use it as a grounding point to return to when you are feeling overwhelmed. What have you created with these hands? What have they touched? Who have they touched? What could you create or achieve with them?

Access the hegu pressure point from traditional Chinese medicine. This is the fleshy point between your thumb and index finger. When stimulated properly this releases beta- endorphins, reducing pain and tension and creating a sense of calm. Look it up on YouTube to learn the technique, it's very easy.

You can also just rub your hands together to warm them up, then place them over your eyelids for a minute.

You could do a three-point check-in—relax and open your jaw, unclench your hands, drop and roll your shoulders. Pair this check-in with something you're already doing so it becomes a new habit—say whenever you go to the toilet, open the fridge or pick up your keys.

Invest in a spiky ball, a foam roller or even just a tennis ball. Learning to massage yourself is one of the greatest gifts you can give yourself. Look for tense spots in your neck and shoulders and lean into how it feels to apply different levels of pressure.

Dance. Move your body in whatever way feels good. It can just be shaking it off to one song, or going for a short walk. The main thing is to avoid sitting with these huge emotions and bodily sensations and then not allowing discharge. My personal view (which is backed by research[14]) is that you need to move through these big feelings. Sitting with big feelings and only using your thoughts to try to move them is like collecting water in a pond. Sure, in moments of stillness you can sift out the yucky parts and 'refresh' the water, but wouldn't it make more sense to keep the water source moving? Water that flows and moves has more energy, more force and opportunity to shift and change.

SOUND

In terms of sound, music is obvious, but if you don't already have set playlists to calm or uplift you, then experiment with what you like. I regularly remind myself how impressed 16-year-old me would be at the choices we have now. No more taping songs from the radio, no more scrimping and saving to buy a CD. There is truly an abundance of options, so feast on it!

AFFIRMATIONS AND COPING STATEMENTS

Almost every therapy or self-development approach uses some form of affirmations, positive self-talk or coping statements. Affirmations can help keep your brain in the present moment and serve as a 'sticky note reminder' not to subconsciously drift back to the past. So many of your negative, unhelpful and untrue beliefs are second nature to you—so much second nature that you maybe don't even notice them, let alone work on challenging them. They are there, though. They show up in every bad mood, every anxious response and every damaging or self-sabotaging behaviour. What you want to work towards is being aware of them, challenging them and replacing them with helpful thoughts.

Positive affirmations work at a subconscious level to rewrite new neural pathways. You always want to frame them in positive terms and in the present tense. Some ideas to get you started:

'I am strong. I am capable. I can do this.'
'Even though I feel overwhelmed, I trust that I am coping just fine.'

If that's not your vibe, then change it to suit yourself. I actually used to hate affirmations with a passion, probably because a former boss gave me a book of vomit-inducing affirmations with dolphins and faeries as a parting gift. Bleurgh. It's not that I hate those things, they just carry negative connotations and don't light me up.

Even though I love and respect Louise Hay and the path she paved for self-development, I choose to speak only in a way that lights me up (see, that's an affirmation!). When I came back to affirmations in hypnobirthing training, I was initially resistant, thinking they weren't for me, but here's the thing. You don't have to make them fit. Choose what aligns with you—language, images, it's got to feel OK for you. How about:

> 'Fuck what others think. I choose to honour whatever I feel about my birth.'
> 'This is coping. This is me owning my shit and I'm doing so well.'

There are some amazing affirmation cards on the market for badass bitches like yourself. I promise you it doesn't have to feel flowery and yuck.

Another option is audio messages from yourself or loved ones on your phone. The brain is far more likely to trust a voice that's familiar. You could have your partner or bestie leave you a brief audio message on your phone with words of encouragement. Familiar voices of loved ones light up the pleasure centre of the brain and can help us feel connected to our life outside the trauma again.

SMELL

The strongest memory triggers are associated with smell, so you could find an oil blend to put on a tissue and smell in the bathroom when you get a break. Find something unique that has no negative associations and that you could use to create a new association. If you used essential oils through pregnancy and birth you may want to avoid the usual lavender and clary sage blends.

Look at the products you use every day—shampoo, creams, laundry detergents, washing up liquids and so on. Can you one hundred per cent say that all of them light you up? Make you feel you are living your best life? My own coach has taught me that life is too fucking short to use products you don't love. I once bought some revolting liquid hand soap from the supermarket. It was on sale and it came in a big bottle. It was the colour of that gentian violet stuff they used to use on baby's cord stumps, and it stank. It was supposed to be 'wild orchid' or something floral but it smelt chemical and gross. But I kept using it because I had loads of the stuff. Every time I washed my hands, I'd feel guilty or annoyed and it would activate all my trauma stuff around scarcity, buyer's remorse and loads of other emotional crap I didn't need to be thinking about every time I washed my hands.

In contrast, on my first trip to Thailand the hotel I stayed at used lemongrass to scent everything. Whenever I smell real lemongrass in cooking or in shampoo or I burn it in my diffuser I feel lighter. It takes me back to a time with no children, warm weather, nowhere to be and permission to relax.

Scent tells a story, conjures emotions and gets us to buy more. Companies spend huge amounts of research figuring out what their flagship stores should smell like. No doubt you've heard about the trick of baking apples or cookies in your oven if you're trying to sell your house (or appease the person coming to do your property inspection if you're renting and don't want to clean the oven!).

Also, think about your own oxytocin. Maybe you've heard that if you're away from your baby and need to pump breastmilk then you should keep a picture of your baby and a blanket or piece of their clothing with you? It's a hack to get your milk flowing more easily, as many people struggle to express milk when they are at work or away from their baby.

When my husband went back to work that first day and I was left home alone to take care of a tiny human, I was terrified. But I found comfort in wearing one of his old T-shirts. Think about keeping an old 'blankie' of your kids, or your partner's old T-shirt, in the car. Maybe it's not your partner you want to smell but your dog. No judgement. You could also keep an old blanket or toy around.

Maybe it's your doula. In my view, a good doula should find it flattering and not creepy that you want to know what perfume or face cream they use. You can keep a sample of that around to remind you of them. My own doula is a total bloodhound. She has not been shy about making it known that she chooses her scents carefully. She knows the power of scent and wants people to remember it. I think she's used to people saying they want to sniff her when they meet her in real life.

TASTE

What are you doing to delight and energise yourself?

A shot of coffee by all means (exhausted mums' club over here!), but the brain's association with coffee might not always be paired with being calm. Often, it's associated with fatigue and stress.

Think about making a ritual with a special drink or treat. A few mindful sips of a special drink or a bite of a special treat you only have after a birth will build specific pathways in the brain, meaning you'll decompress more easily.

Choose one specific flavour or a unique taste not typically consumed every day in your life. You'll then use this to condition your brain to pair it with feeling alert but calm. Even if you're not a tea person, there are plenty of teas on the market that don't look or taste like tea. You don't have to serve it hot or in a teacup.

The point of all of these exercises is to create ritual that delights you. Our ancestors have handed down some shitty coping strategies. Maladaptive behaviours that we have watched as children and copied before we even knew what the meaning behind them was.

Here is your opportunity to redo all of that. If you watched your own parents binge drinking, standing on scales and deprecating themselves, or engaging in numbing or risk activities, you don't have to carry that box anymore. You get to create a new box of coping tools and hand that down to future generations. What might seem like a silly, meaningless, pointless self-care activity is setting the tone. If you have little kids around, they are watching you, copying you. You can say a million 'I love you's' to your babies every day, but if they don't watch you making time for yourself, delighting yourself and acting with self-compassion it's just another case of 'do as I say, not as I do'.

SIXTH OR 'OTHER' SENSE

Are you ready to go deeper than just serving the senses you can identify? Bring your mind, body and spirit into it. You can be an atheist with no interest in spirituality and still work through these without compromising your values and beliefs here. Generally speaking, the people who say 'hell yes' to working with me have a spiritual side. They value something outside themselves and have a respect for rhythm, ritual and thinking about things quite deeply.

This is the 'entertain the idea that you don't know what you don't know' section. What I'm going to teach you here is a bit of a mash-up of positive psychology, mindfulness, acceptance and commitment therapy, cognitive behaviour therapy and dialectical behaviour therapy.

The first step is to realise that negative or painful emotions are not inherently bad. No matter how happy you are, life is going to throw things at you.

Instead of focusing on avoiding or denying negative emotions, I want you to learn valuable skills for tolerating them without becoming dysregulated, that is, feeling it's too much or you're out of control.

GROUNDING

One useful way of starting to work with difficult emotions is through grounding. For some people, this might literally mean you take your shoes off and connect to the ground or the floor. It might mean touching the edges of the chair, wriggling your toes in your shoes.

I love shoes, and, much to my delight during some family research I discovered that I come from a long line of shoemakers on my mother's side. But in a weird way, shoes sometimes represent too much order and oppression for me. My mother tells me that she never saw my dad's feet until after they were married. To this day, my father still gets around in chunky bushwalking boots, though he barely walks to the mailbox these days. If he's not in shoes, he's wearing slippers. Personally, I hate slippers. I always have. I will wear them in winter, but somewhat grudgingly. I hated being forced to wear slippers as a child, so as an act of rebellion, I spend most of my time barefoot.

One of my daily rituals (that's never really planned, but feels *so* necessary) is to step outside with no shoes on. Even in the rain, in the cold, even if the gravel on the driveway or the scorching sun hurts my feet. For a few seconds, it takes me back into my body. When the kids are fighting, I'm overwhelmed and need to get back into alignment I will just go outside with no shoes on. I take recycling out, pick a quick bunch of herbs or throw scraps to my chickens. Connecting back to the earth and feeling a novel sensation under my feet really helps. I might then silently say some affirmations like: 'I'm OK, I'm safe. Big emotions are OK', and another favourite, 'Crying and tantrums are not a reflection on my mothering'.

If you're not into taking your shoes off, then you might just ground yourself by bringing awareness to your breath. Put your hand on your solar plexus (which is roughly a hand's width down form your belly button) and put your focus on letting your hand rise and fall. There's no need to count, or do anything else in particular, just check in with your centre. How do you feel? What do you need? What happens if you slow down your breath and just notice your hand rise and fall?

ORIENTING

Another skill is orienting. This is reminding yourself or someone else that you're safe and in the here and now. Give your brain the direction that you're not back in the trauma, nor are you trying to project, control or push the outcome of the future. You might literally say to yourself 'It's the year 2020', 'It's June' or 'I'm in my car on a Monday'. It sounds simple enough, right? See if you can catch yourself. Notice how many times you're reliving the past or worrying about the future.

You might then orient your attention to something positive or calming, and describing it. It might be the back of your hand, or something you can see out the window. One of the most effective strategies for coping with a panic attack is to shift your focus from internal to external. Remember that what you focus on, you get more of. So, rather than focusing on what's happening inside your body (breathing fast, heart pounding, feeling sick), you'll gently refocus on neutral things outside your body. Use your other senses to see a blue wall, smell coffee, hear the hum of the washing machine, feel the cotton of your shirt and so on. Keep cycling through things you can perceive with your external senses. This will give your nervous system a chance to slow down and your brain a chance to realise that the threat has passed.

ALLOWING

Then there's the skill of allowing. Yep, here it is again. Simply allowing the emotions and the thoughts. You might close your eyes and say 'I'm allowing …' before whatever the feeling or thought or memory might be. So, it might be 'I'm noticing that I feel fear. I'm allowing fear.' Keep going with whatever comes up and see if you can sit with it rather than trying to get rid of it, deny it or change it.

Start with 20 seconds, then two minutes, and keep building up your tolerance. By practising this in small doses you give the nervous system a chance to build a bigger window of tolerance. If you think of negative feelings like waves, the more you can allow and tolerate them the smaller the waves will get, because you're building tolerance. Flexing your distress tolerance muscle.

While you practise this, you can also be practising labelling emotions. Using the language centre of your brain again activates different experiences. It's a way of validating your feelings. When you learn to describe your feelings with strong descriptors—not just angry, but enraged; not just sad, but devastated—you can also begin to dig to see what's under the surface emotions.

For example, anger is a simple primary emotion but it often is a cover for something else—shame, humiliation, or feeling ignored. Try it and see what you come up with.

COPING STATEMENTS

Affirmations or coping statements that are always framed in the positive are also really helpful. Focus on what you want, not what you don't want. Your subconscious doesn't understand the words 'don't' or 'try'. Frame your statements exactly as you wish them to be.

'I am OK', 'I will get through this', 'I can cope'. Again, if we look at trauma research, it's often the people who are able to remain hopeful and focused on what they *do* want who cope better.[13] Please be reminded here that trauma didn't happen because of something you did or didn't do. Using coping statements and believing in yourself and your ability to get through anything will help, but don't use them against yourself. Birth trauma can still happen even if you've got great affirmations and loads of self-belief.

COPING PLANS

Now that you've got a handle on some basic skills for regulating emotions, let's look at how to translate these skills into a safety or coping plan.

SAFETY PLANS

Fun fact about me and my training: I originally trained as an expert in self-harm, suicide and borderline personality disorder. Isn't it funny how sometimes you take a detour in life and think 'Oh, why did I do that?'. Completing a PhD in this area was the perfect training for understanding people and helping them deal with even the most complex and extremes of emotions. It also taught me so much about the mind–body connection and pain.

There are lots of coaches in the world who think they can handle anything a client brings to them without any real training or experience to back it up. I've done the work. I know how to help soothe super-distressed people. Of the time I've spent with people struggling with huge emotions, impulsivity and suicidal ideation, a large part is spent making coping or safety plans. These are basically lists of things the client will do and people they will contact, instead of committing suicide, overdosing or self-harming.

A distressed brain can't problem-solve effectively and a brain which is in active trauma time cannot properly access all its memory systems. Nor can it learn or retain new information. Everyone needs a coping plan. Even if you can't resonate with feeling so overwhelmed that you'd seriously hurt yourself, think about times when you've been overwhelmed. So overwhelmed that you couldn't easily think of something to do to soothe yourself.

Maybe think back to the time you first left the hospital with your brand-new baby (if that's relevant to you). Those thoughts of 'Shit … are they really just going to let me take this baby out into the world? Don't they know I have no fucking idea what I'm doing?'. Maybe it was the first time you were all alone with your baby in the house without your partner or someone else for support. The week before my husband left me with not just one but two kids to look after all on my own while he went back to work, I was so anxious. It didn't matter how many times I tried to reassure myself that people have been doing this for years. The logistics of how I was going to get through a whole day with a newborn and a toddler was just so overwhelming. What helped was having a plan. Some people I knew I could call. Some rehearsal of tasks I hadn't yet performed ('How the fuck do I get two kids into a car by myself?!' and 'How do I take a toddler to the potty in time if I have a baby on me?') and some quick things I could do to feel better if everything went to shit.

Your Coping Plan

Let's start with the three people you're going to call. I want you to think about this carefully. I honestly believe that we cannot expect to have all of our needs met by one person. Not your partner, not your mum, not your best friend and definitely not your baby!

THE CASE FOR HAVING A PROFESSIONAL

Your family and friends are not always going to be real with you. They love you and so they are often going to tell you what they think you want to hear. With people who are familiar to us, we're also in the habit of just off-loading without first checking in. We don't check to see if they are fully present and attending, well-rested, fed and can hold space for us. In our heightened emotional state, we can then feel defensive, shameful, angry or apologise if we notice signs that are reflective of the former. People who are distracted, overtired or hungry, or have a full bladder, are not good listeners. You can be setting yourself up for disappointment if the person you want support from is not able to fully step into the role in that moment.

They may also not be equipped to cope with all the details, or you how you express them, and you may actually traumatise them. Even great listeners often respond with a style of communication that's conditioned, without actually considering how it's helpful, or why they respond that way.

CRYING

Many people might argue that going to touch someone who is crying is an intuitive behaviour. Just what you're supposed to do if you have a heart. This is actually a learned behaviour, and placing your hands on someone can actually prevent them from completing a healthy and needed trauma response. I'm not talking about children here. Let's be clear that there's absolutely nothing wrong with seeking touch when you're a child. It shows empathy and it's a sign of secure, healthy attachments when we seek physical comfort in times of distress. Children also have very underdeveloped nervous systems and need our assistance of physical touch for healthy brains.

I'm not saying don't hug people. I'm talking about those interactions with another adult where someone starts to cry and you feel the need to 'do' something. Perhaps because you're uncomfortable. Perhaps because you've been taught that touching them means reassurance and worth and that not doing anything means you're unfeeling and cold.

Psychologists seldom use touch, but if someone is crying—even the Oprah cry—I wouldn't touch them. It's not just about legalities and covering my arse, it's a way of communicating and allowing. 'I allow this reaction. I accept you. I trust your body to complete this response.'

If I were teaching you to surf, and every time you were about to fall off the board, I caught you, then your body would never learn to figure out how to not fall. I'd also be teaching you that I don't completely have confidence in you. Maybe I need you to need me to save you every time?

If you ever attend a circle, you'll see powerful examples of just being with people in their discomfort and how healing this can be. Not to be fixed, guided or coached. Just accepted as whole, beautiful and complete—even if they have snot running down their face.

Mirror neurons are powerful. When you see an example of someone demonstrating a skill you want or a way of being (whether you're conscious of it or not), your brain will work to have the same brain signals fire, just as a baby learns to use a spoon by watching you.

Trust someone to steer their own ship and let waves naturally find their ebb and flow. Without help.

Crying can also relieve tension. You know how sometimes you get really angry and then you just need to cry? For no particularly reason, you just need to release tension. Toddlers do it all the time. Often, we race in to ask what's wrong, try to fix the problem or chastise the toddler for it because it's uncomfortable and annoying. But as beings who hear 'no' thousands of times a day and have very few autonomous choices with their own bodies and their worlds, they get very tense and frustrated.

Crying allows big emotions and nervous system responses to shift. When people see and feel that they can do this on their own it builds confidence. By rushing in to help you might be blocking an important opportunity. With trauma reactions, women are often taught to suppress anger and instead access sadness or grief. Men are taught to turn off grief and sadness ('boys don't cry') and with nowhere for the charge to go, they express it as anger. We've all got blocked emotions.

We need a chance to access the very emotions that we've been blocking, controlling, deflecting and soothing.

> At this point, check in with yourself. Is there an emotion
> you've been blocking, denying, distracting yourself from and
> not fully expressing?

Have a think about it. What's stopping you? Do you fear your own rage? Or fear the shame and guilt that might come with admitting you're angry at your own baby?

Just watch what comes up. Wait. Sit with acceptance and love for yourself and see what happens.

You need someone who can hold a version of you—the best version of you—in mind so that you can talk without censoring yourself. So that they won't judge you if your phrasing wasn't sensitive, if you need to vent, if you're coming across as judgemental. This is *so* important if you also have weird thoughts that are freaking you out. Weird thoughts are normal, as I'll explain below.

WEIRD THOUGHTS

We all have weird thoughts. Really, honestly, we all do. Take a breath and some comfort in knowing you're not alone if you're only just learning this for the first time. We all have seriously weird thoughts. Some of us simply have more awareness of them and give them more attention than they deserve. Every single one of us has weird thoughts, and probably thousands of them a day. They even have a technical name: ego-dystonic thoughts.

I know Freud didn't always deliver the most feminist, empathic or human-centred ideas, but one of the most reassuring concepts I've ever learned can be credited to him. I can tell you the day, month and year that I first learned this concept. It was Friday afternoon. My lecturer, who seemed way too young to be teaching me, yet so smart and so cool, was wearing a red harlequin print jumper and Buddy Holly glasses. He and his wife has just had a baby, so his commitment to staying awake and keeping his students awake on a Friday afternoon was impressive. In a nutshell (OK, my bad shrink puns will end here) we have two types of thoughts:

1. Ego-syntonic thoughts are the ones that are consistent with or acceptable to our ego. They can be boring thoughts like 'I need the toilet', 'I might go get a sandwich' or pleasant thoughts like 'that's a cute baby'.

2. Ego-dystonic thoughts are ones that are inconsistent with, or unacceptable to, our ego. The ones we'd rather not share. Ever. The ones you think you will take to your grave because living with the secret shame is better than possibly being taken to the loony bin.

Everyone has these weird ego-dystonic thoughts, it's a matter of awareness, frequency and what meaning you put behind them. They are very, very common in new parents. Here is the part where I will reveal some of mine, so that you don't feel as alone or as weird about yours:

'What would my body sound like crashing against the rocks?' (Thanks, Björk!). I've often had a slightly morbid fascination with cause of death. If you fall off a cliff, yes you die, but what exactly is the cause of death? I once pondered a career in forensics but I thought I'd get bored being in a lab all day. Besides, I'm really more interested in the question of what makes you want to jump.

'What if I drown my baby?' All through my postgraduate studies I used to have a recurring dream about drowning things. Our pet guinea pig, our dogs and random babies. I'll add here that the case of Andrea Yates (a mother in the US who drowned her children) was frequently in the news throughout my time at university and it took my fascination. When my babies were tiny, I frequently had dreams about accidentally drowning them, and I sometimes felt anxious during bath time. I think it's no coincidence that many parents describe the postpartum and early parenting period as 'feeling like I'm drowning'. Giving meaning and emotion to thoughts (particularly distressing ones) and telling yourself not to do so seems to have the effect of telling your brain to produce more of them (ironic process theory).[15]

Before I even had children another one of my weird thoughts was that the nail clippers in my drawer were going to fly out and I'd accidentally cut my eyelids. Why did I have this thought? No idea. But it was disturbing enough the first time that I clearly told my brain to not think about it, thus producing the opposite effect where my brain popped up that thought every time I went near that drawer. Again, once I added babies and sleep deprivation to the mix, my new thought was 'What if I'm using these teeny tiny nail clippers and I cut my baby's finger off?'.

Look for it and you'll notice children are way more open and expressive with their ego-dystonic thoughts—until we teach them to suppress them, and perhaps feel shame about them.

I remember once asking my mum in the car 'What would happen if you put a pin in a frog when it's all puffed up? Would it pop or splatter everywhere?'. I remember her looking concerned and telling me it would hurt the frog very much and that we don't do that. I had no intention of hurting frogs, it was just a naturally curious question, asked at what was probably a really bad time. I don't judge my mum for her reaction, because I'm now in that phase right now with my four-year-old. Sometimes, she will just say really off or seemingly insensitive sorts of things that catch me off guard. There is a *huge* difference between a child (or an adult for that matter) expressing a thought and acting on it. A child who expresses curiosity about the experience of killing is not at all the same as the child who actively seeks to torture and kill, and potentially feels little or no empathy about it.

I remember the shame and embarrassment I felt in that conversation about the frog. Many people may have similar memories attached to early childhood questions about sex, bodily functions or body parts. We learn quickly that there are things you are not supposed to talk about. Remember the pink elephant analogy I used earlier in the book, about how rebellious the brain is when you tell it not to do something? You start to see why our brains hang onto thoughts and ideas we'd rather not have.

Having weird thoughts is normal. It doesn't necessarily mean you have a diagnosable mental health condition. It doesn't mean you are a serial killer. Such thoughts tend to pop up when we're exhausted, hormonal, emotional and vulnerable. However, it's like feeding seagulls: the more attention you give them, the more you try to make them mean something, the more the thoughts are likely to increase.

What helps is acknowledging the thought ('hello, weird thought'). Thank your brain and then file it under junk information. Not every single thought we have is meaningful or profound. Our brains produce an awful lot of junk thoughts, just as computers and other devices display weird error messages or surprise us with strange bugs.

Despite what I've just said, if you're really worried, or afraid you'll act on your thoughts, or they are interfering with your day-to-day life, it might mean you could use some extra support.

When you're highly anxious and sleep-deprived and have good awareness of your inner world, weird thoughts can seem worse. If you've struggled with depression, anxiety and suicidal thoughts then they can seem worse. If you've experienced any unwanted sexual experience in your life, it can amplify distressing thoughts. I've heard them all.

'What if I touch my baby's clitoris when I'm wiping her? What if it stimulates her? What if it hurts her? Oh God, am I a sexual predator? Why am I thinking this? What's wrong with me?'

I've heard many, many clients struggle with these 'take it to my grave' kinds of thoughts, but they often don't leave the therapy room. When one of my podcast guests, Doula Rachael Rose, shared that she had these thoughts after the birth of her daughter I think she helped an awful lot of people. When you voice some of the thoughts out loud, they lose their power over you. When you voice your thoughts, you allow other people to breathe into the relief that is realising you are truly not alone.

If the thoughts are constant and are preventing you from being able to live life as you would like, please don't try to will them away on your own. If these thoughts get intense and frequent and/or are accompanied by 'safety behaviours' like having to wash your hands repeatedly, repeating phrases or actions to 'prevent' the bad thing from happening ('compulsions'), this can be a sign of obsessive-compulsive disorder.

Find someone who understands the ins and outs of weird thoughts. Google psychologists who have experience in perinatal psychology and/or obsessive-compulsive disorder. You may not have obsessive-compulsive disorder, but someone who is experienced in that area is potentially going to be a safe person for you to reveal your thoughts to. A huge concern of new parents is that expressing thoughts of harm to themselves or their baby means child protective services will be called and their baby will be taken. There is a *huge* difference between having thoughts and acting on thoughts.

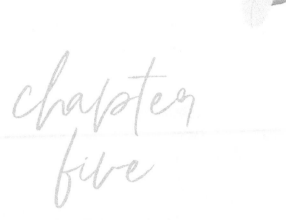

Where Is This Village Everyone Talks About? Social Support

How many times have you heard 'It takes a village to raise a child'? Where is this village? Did I miss the invitation? Actually, that did happen to me with my first ever mothers' group session. Half of us didn't show up to the first session and the organisers realised they hadn't sent out all the invites.

Doing things on our own, in isolation, has become the new Western normal for parents, and it hasn't done us any favours. In theory, I have a much better life than my ancestors. I have a bigger house, more security in finances and health, and yet I think my Scottish ancestors would think that the way I live is really daft.

My parents emigrated to Australia in 1968, but before that generations of people on both sides of my family lived in either Glasgow or Paisley. My ancestors were poor. They lived and worked in crowded conditions and would rarely have been alone. I live in a four-bedroom house with just my husband and two young kids. We live rurally, so my husband commutes for work and I'm alone to parent for at least 12 hours most days.

When I researched my family history, which was around the same time I was researching birth, I was surprised to discover that birthing in a hospital was a relatively new thing. Before my parents came to Australia, as far back as I can find, everyone else in the family was Scottish, with a few Irish thrown in. Before I gave birth, I had somewhat snooty and preconceived ideas that people in my family must have birthed at home because they were poor and couldn't afford a hospital. Little did I know how few of my ancestors might have survived had their parents decided to birth in Victorian and post-Victorian hospitals. Yikes.

We were not wealthy or educated people. Most of my ancestors worked as house servants or labourers or in the cotton mills. Babies died of things that babies should not die from, like gastroenteritis and typhoid from rat bites. There are census records that don't match up, where deceased children are not declared, or children go missing. I cannot imagine the shame those freezing, hard-working women must have felt when the local census taker turned up on the doorstep asking nosy questions about how many babies they'd had.

There are stories of children working in poor houses from as young as seven, and families who reused the name 'John' or 'William' up to three or four times. It wasn't at all unusual for families to have a boy, name him John or William, and then when he died, reuse the name for the next son. Scottish naming traditions used to be quite rigid, following a clear set of rules. What seems morbid to us now was simply our ancestors clinging to tradition.

Birthing at home is a beautiful tradition that has been lost to fear and patriarchy. Less than 100 years ago, most mothers in Scotland birthed at home in their parents' home, surrounded by aunts, cousins, grandmothers and so on. Only after about 12 months or so would a couple then move into their own dwelling with their baby, and that house would only be a few streets away at most. Many of my ancestors also lived with boarders, usually other young women who worked at Paisley's cotton mill or as servants. From an anthropological and historical point of view, we know that the way many of us choose to live now—with so much space and independence—is actually pretty weird. The idea that you might trust a man who has never given birth over your own mother, sister and aunts would seem pretty weird.

Whether the idea of homebirth and family-led care delights or terrifies you, I raise it because I think we have lost a lot of sacred tradition. I still have weekly conversations with psychologists who work in public health about how bizarre it is that we still haven't got enough of the practical side of perinatal mental health services right. We offer therapy sessions during business hours, not accounting for school runs, traffic, parking and having no-one to look after the baby. Childcare within the system that's supposed to be supporting parents often doesn't exist. Parents are asked not to bring their baby to sessions and staff are told not to help mums with prams or feed their parking meters because of occupational health and safety guidelines or because it's seen as crossing a professional boundary. The teenage mum who goes back to school can now no longer attend her therapy appointments because they're only offered during school hours. We've tried to force babies to fit into our hours and our systems and it's clearly not working.

Think about it. We have wine, fast food and even homewares available to us 24 hours a day and yet there's next to nothing open for support during those witching hours. Those hours when babies scream and parents are frazzled, so people get overwhelmed. The times when we could be preventing a crisis and stepping in to help before people end up being admitted to mother-and-baby units in hospitals. Let's also not forget that many hospitals don't even have a mother-and-baby unit, or if they do, it's part of the general psychiatry ward. A general psychiatric ward is not the right environment for a new parent with a baby. The absence of a psychiatric illness is also not wellness.

Why are our new parents and babies not the most treasured members of our community? Why do our governments not fund round-the-clock wellness centres for our most valued and yet most vulnerable community members? Where are the spas, massage treatments, relaxation, nutrition and holistic services for birthing women and babies? Where is the funding for all the services that could prevent the need for new mothers to be in psych wards?

BUILDING YOUR OWN VILLAGE

You need someone, or preferably a few people, who hold the same values of growth, positivity and action, and advocacy over inaction and reaction. You need people who are further along than you—in everything! People who have a bigger vision, who are more experienced and can see a version of future you that you can't even imagine right now. You need to be exposed to new levels so you can reach new levels.

Making friends with other parents is not easy. As someone who never really dated (I've been with the same partner since I was 16), I've sometimes found this process desperation-fuelled and awkward. However, when you really home in on your values and your needs in any relationship, it gets easier. I'm often saying to clients about confidence and visibility that it is a practice. You may be afraid of putting yourself out there, being your authentic self and asking a potential new friend to hang out with you. But if you don't let your unique light come out, then your people can't find you. When you dim your light, the ships can't find you in the dark.

MAKE FRIENDS WITH JUDGING AND BEING JUDGED

What also helps with building your connections as a parent is recognising that we are extremely judgemental creatures. Rather than being judgemental about being judgemental, we can learn the practice of accepting and sinking into it. We need judgements in order to thrive and survive, just as Byron Katie says in her book *Loving What Is*. Judgements help us to decide if a substance is safe to eat; judgements help us decide if someone is about to physically assault us, or harm us and our family in some way. Judgements help us quickly decide (though not always rationally) if someone is in the in-group (safe and like us) or the out-group (not safe or too dissimilar).

From an anthropological perspective, we are really only experienced in keeping track of about 150 other people.[16] This is sometimes referred to as Dunbar's number. British anthropologist Robin Dunbar[17] proposed that humans can comfortably maintain around 150 stable relationships. Everything else becomes noise, so to speak. So, when groups of parents get together and become judgy (either silently or vocally), this is often a reflection of two things. One is that our sleep-deprived brains are looking for tabs to close to make the work of coexisting with other people easier. Messages that are confusing or take too much processing are typically pushed out or ignored by our brains. We move towards things that make sense and away from things that are confusing.

While you make quick judgements about another parent's choices around food, sleep, toilet training, education and discipline, what your brain is really doing is quickly trying to decide if this choice is easy to understand and consistent with your values. If your brain decides that their messaging is too confusing or threatening, you will move your attention away from it. As an example, I was once told a story about a mum who went to her local mothers' group catch-up with her one-year-old. It was snack time for the kids. She pulled out a package of biscuits and offered them around. One mum said 'Thanks, but we don't do biscuits'.

You will likely have an opinion about what you think of that response, quickly drawing on your values, your experiences and beliefs. There's no right or wrong, it's simply an exercise in showing how we quickly deduce things like 'Is this person like me or not like me?', 'Do we have the same values, goals and beliefs?' and ultimately 'Is this someone I want to invest in having in my tribe?'. It's just a biscuit, right? You probably have friends who do biscuits and those who do not. It's wonderful and enriching to surround yourself with people who think differently, isn't it? Absolutely, but when you're an exhausted parent your brain will take short cuts to decide how much you have to invest.

For the most part, we tend to stay in a bubble with people who roughly have the same values, political views and beliefs systems because it's simply less brainwork. We receive regular confirmation that we are 'right' and that we are accepted. There's more harmony and synchronicity when people in a group generally agree. Keep in mind, though, that too much agreement and not enough individuality is how groupthink happens. There was a famous experiment (the Asch conformity experiments)[18] where someone was shown two sticks that were clearly not the same length. Everyone in the group except for the test subject was told to say that they were indeed the same length. So, what typically happened was that test subjects would agree with the group, and say the sticks were the same length, even if deep down they knew that they were not. You might have found yourself in a group where everyone had an elective caesarean section because that's what everyone else in the group did. Or you own a certain brand of pram simply because everyone else in your friendship group did. We can get caught up in our bubble and forget that there's a world beyond it. The most extreme example of this I've seen is when a client once said to me 'But everyone takes heroin at some point, don't they?'. In his bubble, that was true.

The second thing that happens with judgements is that they are an opportunity to examine ourselves. Is this thought even true? Why is it our business? Why do we care? Why do we have to be right? Are we 100 per cent flawless in this area ourselves? Let's say I would like my children to whine less, so I tell them they should stop whining (which I do, regularly). Now, am I a saint when it comes to whining? Do I never complain? Nope. So, while I am attempting to raise decent humans, I also need to be careful of not judging them and demanding expectations of them that I am unable to meet myself.

The subject of child discipline is a good one here, particularly when it's combined with time, Golden Age thinking and the fundamental attribution error. So, imagine if you will the scenario where a toddler is doing what toddlers often do best in supermarkets and having a massive tantrum. In the shop there's often one person who either (a) has raised kids but is remembering through a filter, or (b) doesn't have kids but who definitely has an opinion about the tantrum. You know where this is going, right? Speculations about how things used to be or how things would be if said person was in the same situation. Except that they are not in the past or the future, we're in the present.

The fundamental attribution error is when you judge the acts of other people based on character, but assume that people will magically attribute your acts to the situation and not to your character. For example, if it's someone else in the supermarket, the judgement might be on the parent and the child ('Look at that slack mother letting her child scream!'). However, if it were you in the situation then you'd assume (or rather hope) that other people will judge it by the situation ('They'll see I look tired,' or 'They'll be able to tell my son has autism and be kind.'). Another example is if you are driving and someone suddenly overtakes you, speeds or is driving erratically, you may think 'What an idiot. They shouldn't have a licence. I hope they get booked.' However, if you are the one behaving erratically on the road, you hope others somehow know that your child just had an accident, or you've had a call from your mother's nursing home to say that she's dying, or that you have dreadful diarrhoea and are hoping not to shit yourself in the car.

Judgements and parenting go hand in hand. Having an awareness of this, and what purpose it serves, can make the process of seeking social support and making connections easier. Parenting is a great time to get really clear about your values. What do you believe and what do you stand for? If you can't shine a beacon on those values, people who are potentially perfect members for your village cannot find you.

HOW TO FIND A VILLAGE

When I moved to the countryside at six months pregnant, I didn't know a soul who lived here. I was forced to find people. Truthfully, I didn't bother until I'd already given birth. I started with what I was interested in. There was a mum and bub yoga class in my town, so I went to that. All the people I met were nice, but it took three rounds of classes before I met someone who said 'Let's get a coffee after'. I joined an attachment parenting group on Facebook— and then took over the admin role when a fight broke out about vaccinations. Once I started back at work and word got out that I was the local hypnobirthing teacher and psychologist, I made a few friends that way. A lot of my hypnobirthing clients made instant friendships in classes. Many of them were tree changers just like me who had moved to the area and were looking for new parent friends who shared similar interests and values. I remember sitting in my lounge room with one of my final hypnobirthing classes while we drank kombucha, and discussed local farmers' markets. I laughed with delight and said 'Look at us, we're a cliché!' Alternative-type people who drink kombucha and are into hypnobirthing and organic farming are my people. They may not be your people! But you will find them. Go back to what really lights you up. What are you passionate about?

Other friends of mine go to kangatraining (exercising with your baby in a carrier) or the gym that has a creche. There are music classes, babywearing groups, library sessions, swimming classes and playgroups. Maybe just choose one and see how you go. If there's no parent's group already set up in your area, ask your maternal and child health nurse.

Another option is hiring a postpartum doula, someone to help with the baby, make you food, do washing and keep you company. If you don't have that nurturing family member to step in and help you then you can create one. Doulas are also typically warm people who love connecting families. Even if you don't hire one, you might find that they are happy to connect you with other parents in your area.

THE TYPES OF PSEUDO-SUPPORT TO WATCH OUT FOR

If you look at the people in your circle and don't feel inspired then you don't have a circle you have a cage
—NIPSEY HUSSLE

I call this pseudo-support because I think it's actually pretty common to have interactions with people that may seem OK at the time, but it's not until you're reflecting later that you think 'I actually feel worse now'. When you're a new parent and you're making an effort to talk to other adults, it's easy to second-guess your own reactions, blaming yourself for not being present. Thinking you were just too distracted with the baby, or you're 'too tired' or 'hormonal' when in actual fact, it was the other person who wasn't being all that supportive.

The truth is that there are some people in your life who are going to want to keep you small and feeling stuck or unhappy. Your success, growth and happiness actually make them uncomfortable and defensive. They prefer it when things in your life are difficult, because that's where their comfort zone lies.

Why would anyone want this for you (or themselves?).

1. They enjoy drama and are addicted to negativity and complaining.
2. They are uncomfortable with or unable to celebrate you and find gratitude.
3. They are overidentifying with a victim mindset. I suffered and therefore I want and expect you to suffer too. This happens *a lot* with childbirth stories. Note this is not the same as sharing pain and finding common ground. This is about wanting to constantly stay in the vortex of negativity.
4. They have habits and deeply ingrained childhood and family patterns that equate 'attention' and receiving social support with drama. Some people find it difficult just to pick up the phone and say 'hey, I miss you'. There needs to be some drama. They have learned that in order to receive the attention and support they want, they need to amp up the seriousness or create chaos. Maybe it's the family member who says 'I've got cancer' instead of 'I had a mole removed'.
5. They confuse worry with preparation and pity with compassion.

Think about your boundaries and how you feel with different people in your life. Is there give and take? Avoid people who are going to offer you little other than a tut-tut and a 'poor you'.

PITY

In her books, Gabby Bernstein talks about how pity brings the mood down. It's so true. People can express sympathy and empathy, but when it turns to pity it is disempowering. It grates on you pretty fast and it can mean that you just start putting on a brave face or lying to people.

In the thick of sleep deprivation with both my babies I learned that people were understanding before the six-month mark. Once we were past 12 months, I could see people felt at a loss as to know what to say. Every time people would mean well and ask 'How is she sleeping?' and I basically said nothing had changed, I always received a mixture of unsolicited advice and pity. So I started to lie to people or change the subject. As well as being exhausted and feeling like a failure because I couldn't get my kids to sleep, one of the things I hated most was the pity.

When I met my friend Meg at yoga and learned she also had a baby who was a shit sleeper, it was the best. We'd whine, drink wine, moan, share stories of how people didn't get it and always just express a 'that's sucks' to each other. Each of us was firm in how we wanted to handle things and what worked best for our families. No 'Have you tried ...?', no 'poor you', no looking for magic bullets. Just conversation that always came back to the idea of loving what is. Again, it's a phrase from Byron Katie. You should read her book. It's full of lessons about the beauty of accepting what's in front of you in the present moment, not wishing it was different, trying to force the outcome, but loving what is. Remember you don't have to like it. Accepting that struggle is normal and unpleasant sensations are a part of being a dynamic human is something to always return to.

VENTING

You will have those people in your life: all they do is vent. Before you know it, you get caught in the whirlwind of venting, and while it maybe seems cathartic at the time, you actually leave feeling heavier. More exhausted, as it achieved nothing and maybe you're even resentful.

I'm not saying don't vent. It can be cathartic, but if this is all you're doing with your support system, how is it serving you? How is it getting you closer to your goals, challenging you to stretch yourself and celebrating you? Too often it's when things are going well that we don't spend any time reflecting or celebrating that.

COMPETITIVENESS

Unfortunately, mothers' groups, playgroups and even online groups dedicated to birth trauma can be prone to competitiveness.

Before I had my first baby, I'd heard so many awful stories about mothers' groups that I had absolutely no intention of going to one. The judginess, the competitiveness. Woman after woman I spoke to (clients, family and friends) all seemed to have similar stories about leaving the group feeling worse or dropping out. I'd heard so many rotten stories I'd actually drafted a book proposal about mothers' group dropouts!

I can't remember why I even decided to go to mine. It wasn't in the same town as me, I barely felt physically OK to drive again and I had no-one around to take me. We'd moved to town in my seventh month of pregnancy and I guess I figured I (a) hadn't made any friends yet, and (b) had to get out of the house at some point.

I was an absolute mess the day of the group. It was stinking hot. I had no idea what to dress the baby in so that she would not overheat, yet keep the sun in the car off her skin and still look like I made an effort. I'd only recently learned to drive, and leaving the house by myself with a baby in the car was slightly terrifying. I was anxious about whether to put makeup on to make myself feel better, or whether that would make me look 'too together'. Every microscopic decision seemed fraught with fears of being judged either way. I wasn't breastfeeding but expressing breastmilk and giving it to Stella in a bottle. I was convinced that everyone there was going to judge me. I also figured that once they found out I was a psychologist no-one would want to talk to me anyway.

To my surprise, it was actually alright. More than alright. Many people I know are surprised to hear that we're all still friends and see each other. There's genuinely never been any drama. Around half of our group all got pregnant again within the same couple of months, so we just kept hanging out together.

If your group is not making you feel supported, you're having to fake things or come home feeling judged, then it's time to find a new group. Your energy is precious. Don't waste it on people who are draining it.

IF YOUR SUPPORT SYSTEM ISN'T SERVING YOU, FIND A NEW ONE

Don't wait until everything goes to shit to connect with people. Strong social connection is about celebrating the wins, analysing why things in your life are working well so that you can maintain them and catch yourself doing good. It's about the choices you are making that are activating the change—not just good luck or a good year. You are responsible for your own thoughts, behaviours and outcomes. You don't wait until your flowers look dead before starting to watering them.

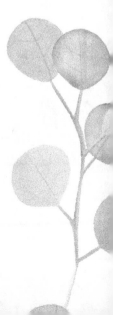

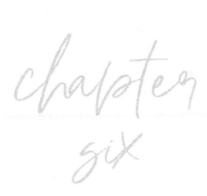

chapter

six

Your Brain Is a 24-Hour Pharmacy: How Hormones Can Be Your Helpers

What if I told you that you already have naturally occurring drugs in your body that are up to 40 times more powerful than morphine?

I don't know why we aren't being taught this stuff at school. Learning about the hormones of birth, stress and relaxation changed my life, so I wanted to include a brief, easy-to-digest section on the power of endorphins for a few reasons:

1. I've found the application of working with your own natural endorphins to be an absolute game-changer in terms of managing health, mood and pain. When you feel like you've struck gold you want to tell the world.

2. If you're planning to birth again, you'll really benefit from this information. No matter what kind of birth you end up with, working with your body's natural hormones will benefit you and your baby.

3. Even if you never plan to birth again, you can use these skills for dentist visits, cervical screening, surgery, or any time you might want to cope with unpleasant sensations or pain.

Synchronicities are a beautiful thing. I've long thought of myself as someone who had a low pain threshold and was a bit of a wuss, really. One of the reasons I studied self-harm for so long and in such detail was because it was so fascinating to me. In the early days, I really couldn't fathom how or why someone would choose to deliberately hurt themselves, so I researched it. Once I understood the psychophysiology (how emotions influence processes like heart rate, sweating and breathing) behind the behaviour, it all made perfect sense as a coping strategy. A maladaptive one, but still a coping strategy. It also made sense of why it's such a difficult behaviour for most people to discontinue. In a nutshell, most people who self-harm feel incredibly anxious, out of body, angry or distressed before they cut. The act of breaking the skin floods the brain with beta-endorphins (which make you feel good and often provide pain relief) and people report feeling less anxious, calmed and relieved.[19] Their heart rate and breathing rate tend to mirror this too.[20] It's like an extreme version of a runner's high. Now obviously this doesn't happen for everyone, but for some it soon becomes a conditioned response and even the mere thought of cutting or picking up a razor is associated with feeling calm.

Jump ahead a few years to me planning for my first birth and wondering how on earth I was going to manage the pain. After initially thinking I'd have all the drugs, I watched the movie *The Business of Being Born*, and soon changed my mind. A friend of mine who was also a clinical psychologist was teaching hypnobirthing, so I thought I'd give it a go. I did more than give it a go: I immersed myself in it and became a practitioner, thinking that if it worked for me I'd teach it as part of my skill set, and if it didn't, I'd move on.

The way that you learn to condition your brain and body to anticipate a calm, positive birth made so much sense. Breathing techniques, acupressure (where you apply pressure without needles), mindset tools, using touch to release endorphins and manage pain—it was all so useful. I don't know about other programs, and I know they vary, but for me the Hypnobirthing Australia program changed my life. The tools and techniques are things I still use today, and I really think they helped make my traumatic births manageable rather than unmanageable.

So, for me, preparing for birth and coping with two traumatic births has had an awful lot to do with endorphins, hormones and understanding the mind–body connection.

What I want to do here is give you an overview of some of the most important hormones and how you can use them for birth (should you choose to birth again) and for managing stress and general wellbeing. Even if you are someone who says 'no, I want all the drugs' there's still some benefit to learning about what's already there for you to work with.

I've had more than one woman in my hypnobirthing classes begin by telling me she's definitely having pethidine, morphine, an epidural or an elective caesarean section. By the end of the course they've changed their minds and gone on to have unmedicated, physiological births. Not because their previous choices were bad or wrong, but because they didn't have all the knowledge; they needed to make an informed decision. They hadn't been taught about just how strong they actually were, or had someone coach them and believe in their ability to do whatever they set their minds to. If you are someone who had all the drugs or wants all the drugs, go for it; I'm just passing on information here.

Even if you're never birthing again, chances are, at some point, you might injure yourself, have surgery, or get run down or depressed. Or you'll know someone who will. Again, it's not about saying 'natural or nothing' here. It's more like looking in the fridge to see what you've already got that's nourishing and will make you feel good before heading off to do a Macca's run. Quick-acting chemicals, whether in food or drugs, might make you feel amazing at first, but then as the effects wear off, you'll often have side effects. Keep in mind here that I'm a psychologist and I also know a bit about hormones and physiology. I'm by no means an expert, so this is just an introduction. Please, do your own reading and speak to your own care providers.

MELATONIN

The dark hormone. There is a reason why babies who arrive on their own terms typically do so in the dark hours. The same is true for other mammals. A domestic cat will usually find a quiet, dark space to birth her kittens.

Melatonin regulates sleep, among other things. Sunlight turns it off, telling your brain to wake up, whereas darkness turns it on. This is partially why you should avoid using devices that emit blue light (TV, phones, computers) two hours before bed.

Melatonin also synergises with oxytocin for uterine contractions during birth. So, if you're in a hospital and it's daylight, one thing you can do is to close the curtains and turn off the lights.

ADRENALINE/NORADRENALINE

Adrenaline, when it's activated at the right time, is super helpful. It stops us from walking in front of traffic, and gives us a boost in the final part of labour. It helps with the natural expulsion reflex to help babies be born.

However, high levels of adrenaline in early labour can inhibit oxytocin production, therefore slowing or stalling labour. Feeling safe and supported is what reduces adrenaline.

CORTISOL

This is the stress hormone. It can be measured in saliva. One of the most terrifying bits of research I've ever seen is how someone (e.g. an infant) can look totally fine and quiet, yet still have high levels of cortisol surging through their body.[21] You don't have to be screaming to be stressed. Cortisol tells your body it's time to fight or flee and it will shut down any other process that's not part of the defence system.

PROLACTIN

The 'mothering' hormone. Prolactin is the major hormone of breastmilk synthesis and breastfeeding. It peaks at night time (usually at ungodly hours) but can help you feel relaxed, and make it easier for you and your baby to sleep. Breastfeeding through the night and activating prolactin is what inhibits ovulation (and periods returning) for many women postpartum.

OESTROGEN, PROGESTERONE AND TESTOSTERONE

Understanding that (premenopausal) women are cyclical is a

game-changer in terms of managing your mood, your energy and life in general.

Having your hormone levels checked postpartum, and throughout your life, is something I'd recommend. I often wonder how many care providers actually check in with this before rushing to diagnose 'depression' or 'anxiety'. As I've mentioned before, this is a really good question for all your care providers: 'How do you know if what I'm experiencing is hormonal or a reaction to lack of sleep or to diet, or if I am depressed for some other reason?'

It can take a really long time for your menstrual cycle to become regular again after pregnancy, birth and breastfeeding. Figuring out what is 'you' and regular or irregular for you after having babies is actually a huge shift in identity. It was for me, anyway.

Even as I write this, it's coming up to 12 months or so since my youngest fully stopped breastfeeding and I still find it difficult to distinguish between 'sleep-deprived', 'premenstrual' and 'I'm actually just sad or pissed off'. Suddenly, my cycles are way shorter than they used to be. I get raging premenstrual syndrome that's worse than it ever was before I had kids. I cry just about every day. After years of tracking my cycle, I'm getting better at anticipating ebbs and flows in energy, but it's an ongoing study, which will change anyway!

People who follow a menstrual cycle tend to match the phases of the moon. Before industrialisation and the introduction of artificial light, women typically menstruated with the full moon and ovulated with the new moon (or vice versa).

Men, on the other hand, tend to have a day-and-night cycle. The balance between pathologising periods and expecting women to function in the same way as men is still not great. There are, however, amazing people advocating and researching for menstrual policies in the workplace. Essentially, it's about acknowledging that at certain times in the month women need to rest, especially if they have heavy, painful periods, migraines or endometriosis.

Women should not have to be pathologised into being 'sick' in order to take a day of rest. Jane Hardwicke Collings and Dr Daniella Arabena are two women I know who have a lot of wisdom to share in this area, and both have been guests on my *Birth Trauma Training for Birth Workers* podcast.

SEROTONIN

We are all programmed to pursue a 'pleasure' hormone, and serotonin is one of them. People who don't feel good will seek out things to stimulate serotonin. Adaptive ways might be things like getting out in the sunshine, moving their bodies, eating gut-healthy foods (serotonin is largely formed in the gut), connecting, meditating and laughter. These are all behavioural things that help buffer us from depression. Less adaptive ways of getting serotonin might be turning to unhealthy foods, relying on caffeine, impulsive behaviours (like constantly picking up your phone) or becoming rigid about exercise and food. At the more challenging end of the spectrum people might turn to drugs and alcohol, risky sex, self-harm and other self-damaging or risky behaviours.

New parents are at risk of serotonin depletion because their focus and their physiology change drastically. There are clear links between lack of sleep, low vitamin D levels, poor eating and low serotonin. When serotonin levels become quite low, we might diagnose someone with depression. Trying all the adaptive ways of creating serotonin in the body naturally is a good practice, but sometimes we need more help. I'm a psychologist who works with behaviours and thoughts to help people with low mood and depression, but there is also a place for antidepressant medication. I advocate a 'natural' approach first, but medication sometimes saves lives. Suicide is still the leading cause of death in new mothers, and if it were as simple as getting some more sunshine and meditating, then we wouldn't have the global health crisis that we do. Please do you, and what you need to do to be well.

BETA-ENDORPHINS

Beta-endorphins are amazing. Put really simply, they are produced in the pituitary gland of the brain and they block the sensation of pain. They are produced in response to exercise, stress and bodily injury. I once went out on a friend's father's boat to a little sheltered cove off Tasmania. I think we collected oysters or mussels, I don't quite recall. But I remember getting back into the boat and my friend's dad saying 'look, your foot is bleeding'. I had no idea. I must have cut it on a shell. Probably my beta-endorphins had kicked in before I noticed. Yet once I saw the blood gushing and paid attention to it, I felt pain. (In hypnosis, we teach people to see the word 'pain' as an acronym for Pay Attention Inwards Now.)

One way to naturally activate your beta-endorphins (without injuring yourself) is to exercise. That runner's high that you may have heard of is a concoction of endorphins. Acupuncture (with tiny needles) is another way to stimulate beta-endorphins.

Acupressure (where you apply pressure to meridian points with your hands rather than needles) is another way. There are pressure points that help with nausea, anxiety, fatigue and pain. One of my favourites in both births was the Cilao (BL-32) point. Essentially it involved my husband jamming his thumbs into the two little hollows in my lower back. It might sound strange, but it was really a life saver! Dr Kate Levett is a wealth of knowledge in this area, and has completed great research (for those of you who are sceptical!). Another person to search for is Debra Betts. She has a range of really helpful YouTube demonstrations on acupressure points for pregnancy, birth and postpartum.

OXYTOCIN

Oxytocin is often called the love hormone, which soothes trauma, deepens relationships and makes birth smoother. If you're calm and not in 'fight or flight' mode, you'll get a big release at the start of labour, when your baby is born and during breastfeeding. Oxytocin is what gets babies in and gets babies out!

Dr Sarah Buckley talks about building up an oxytocin bank before birth. Unlike sleep and the old advice 'Sleep now because you'll need it when they baby comes', you can in fact bank oxytocin. I think this is simply amazing. Even if you're having a planned caesarean section and you're numb from the waist down or don't feel particularly 'loved up', having a store of oxytocin is still (potentially) going to make birth smoother. It makes sense, because where there is oxytocin, cortisol and stress get turned down. Where there is an absence of fear, pain and tension, there is more room for comfort and confidence.

THINGS THAT HELP PROMOTE OXYTOCIN:

Whether you are looking to bond with your partner and/or your baby, or to prepare for birth again, there are loads of things you can do to promote natural oxytocin:

- Light-touch massage
- Stroking and cuddling pets
- Acupressure and acupuncture
- Skin-to-skin cuddles, kissing
- Genital and breast stimulation and orgasm.

Orgasmic birth is totally a thing. You can search for Debra Pascali-Bonaro and her work in this area.

Things that help promote oxytocin after birth:

- Keeping the baby close, spending hours together skin to skin
- Babywearing
- Sniffing your baby. Smell is how your baby first recognises you, and your unwashed breasts and droplets of breastmilk smell the same as the amniotic fluid. Smelling your baby lights up the reward pathways in your brain
- Sniffing your partner's T-shirt
- Having a picture of your baby to look at if you have to express milk when away from the baby. Making a video of yourself sniffing and kissing your baby. (This is handy to watch later to take a trip down memory lane when your two-year-old is screaming bloody blue murder.)

SYNTHETIC OXYTOCIN

Is synthetic oxytocin the same thing as oxytocin? No. Before I studied any independent childbirth education, I'd read plenty of studies using 'oxytocin' to treat psychopathology. I thought the obvious thing to do with birth was to go straight for the synthetic oxytocin, especially if it's the same thing, right?

Synthetic oxytocin is chemically identical to natural oxytocin but it has different effects because it is not released from and within the brain. Syntocinon and Pitocin (synthetic forms) are *not* in practice the same thing as oxytocin, even if it says 'oxytocin' on the box. And yes, that happens, and I can't believe companies can get away with it.

Synthetic oxytocin works in the same way to promote contractions (though they are typically less smooth, more erratic and more intense). Having birthed with and without it, I definitely recall the difference. Contractions from my induction were more intense and less predictable and there was less of a break in between. Manageable, but they didn't feel the same as a birth without Syntocinon. The most important difference, however, is that synthetic oxytocin actually blocks the brain's natural oxytocin (let that sink in). This means that you won't receive any of the loved-up or calm feelings, or you'll have to work harder to feel the good vibes.

Dr Sarah Buckley's book *Gentle Birth, Gentle Mothering* is an excellent reference for more information about hormones in pregnancy, birth and postpartum.

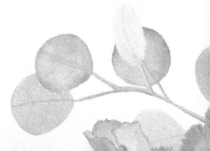

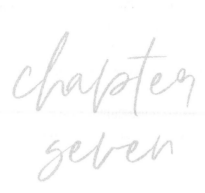

Breath:
The Coping Tool That's Always With You

Fear is excitement without the breath
—FRITZ PERLS

Breath, the coping tool that's always with you. When I was reflecting on what tools I thought were really the most useful to me in pregnancy, birth, trauma, times of anxiety and general life, breath has been fundamental. So fundamental that I've ended up including a whole chapter on it. Breath is the one tool that is lifelong, and when you learn different techniques to maximise your health and wellbeing it really is life-changing. Breathing is what got me through two unmedicated births. Breathing is what has helped me connect with deceased loved ones, spirit guides, creativity, joy, peace and healing.

I remember visiting my husband's grandmother and her husband, whom they called Dore. He was an ex-police officer. A very straight-up-and-down, three-meat-and-veg kind of guy who, at least from my experience, tended to find the negative in most things. He was unwell with a list of various health complaints—gout, arthritis and emphysema. I remember him complaining that he'd been sent off to see a health practitioner to learn how to breathe properly. You can imagine what he thought of this idea. He may have said 'codswallop' or maybe it was 'bullshit'—I can't recall, but the idea seemed to him to be completely ridiculous. 'Why do I have to be sent off to learn to do something I've been doing since I was born?'

Except that effective breath is life and most adults don't breathe correctly. This is something I've observed in every aspect of my practice, as a psychologist, a postgraduate researcher and a childbirth educator. Many of us are not taught how to breathe properly at all or how to interpret our bodily signals. Which is why, at many stages of my practice, I'd end up seeing older guys just like Dore who ended up in the emergency department thinking they were having a heart attack when in actual fact what they were experiencing was a panic attack. They are indistinguishable to most people.

Sure enough, we start out breathing well. You watch a newborn and see how their diaphragm rises and falls with relaxed breathing. Somewhere in early childhood our breathing moves up and becomes shallower. We stop breathing from our bellies and start to breathe from our chests. We have an epidemic of children who are struggling with anxiety and stress as testament to this.

When I was completing my honours, masters and PhD degrees I used psychophysiological methods to collect data. This meant measuring people's heart rate, skin conductance (sweating) and respiration. Of the 100 or more people I took through this process of attaching electrodes and fitting a respiration gauge, only five or so people needed the respiration gauge around their abdomen. And they were usually singers, swimmers or dancers. Everyone else had to have the gauge (a Velcro-like belt) wrapped around their chest in order to pick up a reading. We are primarily a generation of chest breathers.

What I'd like to do in this section is to encourage you to think more about your breathing, and teach you the basics of how to optimise your breath. This is often easier to teach in person, or visually, so I'd encourage you to read over the concepts and then cement your learning with video demonstrations, or find a teacher. An independent childbirth educator, a yoga teacher, a mental health practitioner, a breathwork facilitator or other professional can help.

START WITH YOUR FACE

What are you doing with your mouth right now? Is your jaw clenched or relaxed? We hold a lot of tension in our faces! An interesting fact for anyone who has given birth is that tension in the jaw directly correlates to tension in the pelvis. Yawning, pulling silly faces, blowing raspberries and letting out noises or singing are ways to release tension in the jaw and send the message to your nervous system that it's time to relax.

RELAXATION BREATHING

For someone who is a beginner to the idea of relaxation breathing, a good place to start is to direct your attention to breathing through your nose instead of your mouth. Breathing through your mouth, if you're not mindful about it, can easily lead to hyperventilation and feeling panicked. Taking big gulps of breath through your mouth can trigger your nervous system to go into 'fight' mode.

So, start with taking a long, deep breath through your nose, holding it for a second and then letting it go through your nose again if you can (out your mouth is fine too). From here, there are two quick ways to check in with your breathing.

TWO-HANDED BREATHING

Place one hand on your chest and one hand on your belly. Sit back, breathe as you normally would and see which hand is moving. If you are prone to breathing from your chest, see if you can get the hand on your belly to move instead. Take long, slow breaths in. As you breathe in, your belly should go out like a balloon filling with air. This is diaphragmatic breathing. Many of us were taught that taking a big breath in means your belly should go in too. Many women have also been socialised to 'suck in' our bellies in so as not to look bloated or pregnant. If this is you, I want you to learn to release that idea. Watch a baby, watch a dog. They do not suck their bellies in when they are taking relaxed breaths or sleeping. If you're not pregnant, and it's safe to do so, another thing you can try is lying down and placing a big book on your belly. Your goal is to breathe by pushing your belly out and getting the book to move instead of your chest.

LOCKING AND UNLOCKING YOUR FINGERS

Another method I like to teach is to lock your fingers over your belly. The goal is to take deep breaths in, and as you do, your fingers should unlock. As you breath out, your fingers should naturally lock again.

As I mentioned, a video or in-person demonstration might be easier, so don't lose hope if it's not making sense yet.

If you are planning to birth again, I highly recommend taking an independent childbirth education course that teaches optimal breathing techniques for birth. Relaxation breathing is great for early labour, and in between contractions, but breathing through a contraction and breathing to bear down to birth your baby are different skills.

BREATHWORK

If you're not pregnant, and your healthcare provider indicates it is safe to do so, another approach I recommend is breath work. There are a few different approaches to this technique. I'm not a certified practitioner, so what I'll share here is simply my own experience as a participant.

The first time I went to a breathwork session it was also the first night away from our kids for my husband and me. Because we are those people. Or rather I'm that person and I made him come along. Most people surely go to dinner and a movie. Instead, I wanted deep insights, experiential learning and connection, and to see what all the fuss was about. Several of my coach friends are breathwork practitioners and I also know many people who've said breathwork was amazing for trauma, so off I went.

I attended a two-day workshop with Lukis Mac and Helle Weston from Owaken (previously called the o2awakening). Initially, I was worried that I might pass out or vomit, or both. Having been trained in a discipline that encourages people *not* to mouth breathe, I found going and doing just that for over an hour at a time daunting and maybe even a little dangerous. However, early on in my training I remember being taught that one of the most effective methods of supporting people with hyperventilation and panic is to actually induce it with them—safely, of course, with chocolate, an espresso and a hot stuffy room. Once the light-headed, panicky feelings come, we can then safely support people through the sensations and let the nervous system regulate itself, thereby proving to someone that they can master their own physiology and ride through the panic to the other side where calm is waiting for them.

Truthfully, I've actually never used this approach with a client, but I've accidentally induced that state in myself many times with a strong coffee and a brownie. I'm also that person who likes the idea of a hot bath, takes the time to fill it up and then needs to jump out two minutes later because they're having heart palpitations and nausea.

The first day of the Owaken workshop experience was learning how to work with deep mouth-breathing to experience altered states of consciousness. We did a one-hour guided breathwork journey, and it was intense but exhilarating. I felt all tingly and cold and then I had all sorts of interesting insights and sensations. In that first session I laughed my head off. Full body cackling and tears. It was both a surprise and a delight. While other people around me were having this deep, grief-stricken and traumatic reactions, I was accessing fun and laughter. This is often the missing element in my own trauma work. I will go to the deep, yucky parts but then forget to play. If you are open and receptive to whatever comes out a breathwork session, you'll get out of it what you want to get out of it. Helle and Lukis are very chill and respectful of the fact that not everyone is into spiritual stuff. I am, but my husband is not so much, and he had a completely different experience from me.

It's a difficult experience to describe, but I interacted with spirits and animals and had great fun. I interacted with a 'being' whom I instantly recognised as my son. Yes, the baby I lost to miscarriage at 10 weeks. The phrases that come to mind to describe that interaction are: 'complete shit stirrer', 'thanks for the ride, I was never intending to stay', and 'I just came to fuck shit up for you and remind you that you're not in control'. There's no science or logic for me to default to in order to explain any of this, and that is the point. In that hour, I was able to let go, not take life too seriously and simply live in the moment and play.

Afterwards, I felt exhilarated and starving. My husband and I ate oysters and chips and drank cold white wine on the rooftop bar of our hotel. Within an hour, I learned that two of my friends had birthed their babies, which I somehow already knew. I felt more passionate and purposeful in my values and my relationships. Then I crashed. Getting out of bed the next day was rough, but I went along to experience Level 2.

On day two, we went deeper into Energy Medicine, deep self-enquiry and the Mind–Body connection. We did a bunch of exercises with strangers in dyads or small groups, most of which I'd done before. Eye gazing, sharing hopes and dreams and learning a little about Body Talk. Then we did another 75-minute breathwork journey. This time I struggled a little at first with the experience of trying to force something to happen. I got frustrated that nothing was happening and had to work a bit harder to consciously drop into the experience. This time, instead of interacting with young, playful impish 'beings', I was met with old, crabby crones, one of whom was particularly cranky. She's cranky at me right now as I type this because I can't remember her name! She has visited me before, and my priestess friend has told me she is probably the Celtic goddess Cerridwen. She's keeper of the cauldron, representing the wisdom of old age, and as far as my experience of her goes, cranky as fuck.

Basically, she was fed up with me for whining. Fed up that I turned my back on the ancient family wisdom—women who knew how to use herbs to heal and communicate with animals. Women who had deep knowledge about birth and trauma and healing, before they were burned and drowned. As she poked me with her stick, she said words to the effect of 'For fuck's sake stop whining. All you have to do is click your fingers, and magic will happen'. So, I clicked my fingers. My entire body went tingly. I was surrounded by the presence of a lot of women, just as I had during the birth of my second daughter. They had unfinished business. As I type this now, it's becoming clear to me that I've had some unresolved anger around this birth. I can recall being in the zone, surrounded physically by people I trusted, and metaphysically by these other women when I was interrupted. Learning that I had to change from my all-fours position and go on my back pissed me off royally. From that moment, all of my spirit-type guides disappeared and I was back in the real world.

This second breathwork journey was to resolve unfinished business. There's a South American practice, which also exists in other cultures, called closing the bones or mother roasting. From what I understand, it serves two purposes. One is to physically wrap the birthing woman up with fabric and close the hips, which widen from pregnancy and birth. The other purpose is to call the mother's spirit back into her body. During the shoulder dystocia manoeuvres, and soon after Lily's body left mine, I was not in my body. Instead I was looking down on my body, feeling numb. In psychology, we call this depersonalisation. It's not always a bad thing, for I think that temporarily leaving my own body allowed me to endure the intense sensations of having a five-kilogram baby manually rotated out of my birth canal.

In this second breathwork session, I felt the urge to place my hands on my hips and push them back together. I felt an orb of hot, crackling, surging energy in each hand, just like some supernatural being out of that show, *Charmed*. I alternated between placing my hand on my hips and putting them on my heart and my womb space. They may not have been my hands. Afterwards—just as cranky-pants Cerridwen made the gesture of washing her hands of me—I curtly said 'alright, we're done'. I then desperately needed to pee, so I slowly got up and tried not to trip over people as I made my way to the toilet to do what felt like the biggest wee of my life. I was not at all energised after that second session; I was exhausted and slightly grumpy about having to head home to my children.

As an interesting coincidence, when we arrived home and I'd greeted the kids, I went to go check on my chooks. As I entered the chook house, I saw my favourite hen, a black Brahma, with emerald tinges to her feathers, dead on the floor. There was no sign of illness or attack. She most likely had a heart attack, or she fell. It happens. Chickens are susceptible to sudden deaths from completely unpredictable circumstances. I share this because this is exactly what happened before I birthed Lily. We went out for the day, I got my hair done for the last time, and I went to close the chickens up. The top chook, a sassy pants non-cuddly hen named Ruby, lay dead on the floor. It was the first time I had ever had to deal with a dead hen, and I was devasted. No signs of illness or injury, she looked like she literally just dropped dead. The day I finished writing this book, another one of my hens, Maya, died.

Hens, of course, represent the archetype of the mother and child. Nurturing and self-sacrifice. Hens symbolise female fertility, birth, children and sexuality. They also represent something significant happening in your life.

There's no research that I'm aware of for breathwork being used for birth trauma. What I'm giving you here are my personal insights and opinions, which of course may or may not suit you. However, I've personally found this approach so useful, and as someone who is extremely analytical and often in my head, I found it a welcome surprise for finding insight and healing.

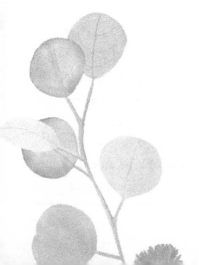

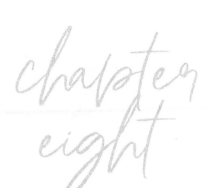

What Is a Debrief and Do You Want or Need One?

A popular idea that gets discussed in the same breath as birth trauma is the idea of a birth debrief. In Australia at least there's no real clear consensus on what that is, who is skilled to do it or if it's even helpful. I've put this section together to answer some of the common questions and help you decide if you want one, and what it might look like.

What is a debrief? It depends who you ask. A debrief might mean any of the following:

1. an informal chat
2. an introductory or stand-alone counselling session
3. a review of your birth notes
4. guidance about how to make a complaint or begin legal proceedings
5. gaslighting. A meeting which is called a 'debrief' but where other people do most of the talking. The tone is defensive rather than actually supportive and

the intention is to fob you off and avoid blame and litigation.

Let me outline what I think a debrief should be.

Psychological debriefs became the gold standard for a while after critical incidents—natural disasters, shootings and other major events. We assume we need to ease people's distress and to prevent it getting worse. It makes sense, but here's the thing: the evidence is mixed.

Some claim that a debrief is helpful; others claim it doesn't really do anything, but at least does no harm. Others claim that it does do harm, and actually increases the risk of people developing long-term psychological symptoms. Suffice it to say the evidence is mixed.

A birth debrief isn't quite the same as critical incident debriefing. For one, it should just be the birthing woman and her partner or support person. It's about active listening and sharing. Maybe that's going over birth notes with a care provider, but that would depend entirely on the birthing woman.

Going over the birth with the midwife or obstetrician (if possible) might be helpful, but there are some questions to consider first:

Do you feel completely safe and supported by this person? If you felt they were rude, unsupportive or let you down in some way during the birth, then it's possible these feelings will come up again in a debrief. If they do, you may end up feeling unheard and unsupported. You could come away from a debrief feeling like nothing has changed, or you feel worse.

Is this person going to have to censor themselves in some way? Is it reasonable to expect that they can give you their authentic reaction? Or, do they need to consider hospital policy, their insurance policy wording and unofficial 'rules' in what they say?

For example, an all-too-common scenario in birth might be that your midwife was overruled by someone else. Maybe you were birthing beautifully, fully supported by a midwife and then an obstetric registrar came in and decided that an intervention (such as a caesarean section) was needed. Was your midwife actually going to be able to say 'yes, I'm pissed off with that decision too!'.

Just recently, I was supporting a childbirth educator whose hypnobirthing client had a rough outcome. The midwife supporting her—who may have been coming off a double shift—was tired and communicated this to the birthing mum by saying words to the effect of 'I'm too tired. I don't think I'm making good decisions so I'll hand you over to someone else'. While it's good to recognise this in yourself, and make changes, using this wording with a client is so damaging.

This is why an independent party like a psychologist or counsellor, someone not employed by the hospital where you birthed, might be a better choice for a debrief.

You don't have to be a counsellor to be a good listener, but I would at least want to know that someone has insight and awareness into their listening blocks. Every single one of us has them. True listening—where you are fully attending to someone else—is a practice. Most of us are still guilty of interrupting, talking over the top of people, rehearsing our answer, defending or even just parroting. It's human to become distracted by the fact that you need a wee, your stomach is rumbling, or you're trying to take a peek at the clock.

I love that quote about listening to your children as if they are the wisest beings on the earth, but I can't do it all day. I especially can't fully attend when the conversation is along the lines of 'poo poo bum bum, I did a fart'.

Pure listening and empathising is hard work. Actually, to put it bluntly, it's draining as all fuck. You need really good boundaries around your empathy. You need energy. You need to be skilled at stillness—for example, waiting until the right time to shift your body in case this movement interrupts the flow of ideas or your client interprets this as boredom, discomfort or disapproval.

Sometimes, people offer debriefs out of a need to 'do something' because it makes them feel useful. Sometimes they feel pressured to say something meaningful sand insightful so they resort to clichés, bargaining or trying to rebut or reframe your experiences.

I'm wary of phrases like:
> 'the main thing is ...' (Why does there need to be a main thing?)
> 'at least you've got a healthy baby'
> 'but...' (Saying 'but' after someone has expressed an emotion is not truly listening and putting their needs first.)

'it's just ...' (as in 'It's just a second-degree tear')
'I understand exactly how you feel.' (How could you possibly? You're not the same person and you've not lived the same life!)

There's loads more, but the point I'm trying to get across is that a debrief is about you, and how you feel. You should feel safe, free to say what you need to say and not filter, defend or overexplain yourself.

There really isn't any need for the person doing the debrief to 'do' anything. You're not broken, you don't need advice. You need a container to feel seen, heard and validated. To feel that you matter and someone gives a shit not just about the baby, but about you.

I would want you to hear lots of:
> 'Of course you feel that way.'
> 'That sucked.'
> 'You're coping the best you can.'
> 'I can see how strong you are.'
> 'I totally acknowledge that.'
> 'You are a rock star!'

These are just examples. It's not an exact script!

Despite the reservations I've mentioned, a debrief can also be helpful. For one, it's a way of communicating that this is an event worth talking about. I never, ever want birthing women to think that there's just nothing you can do after a traumatic birth. If someone is offering you an opportunity to talk about your experience and it feels good in your body to do so, then go for it.

Our midwives, doulas, nurses and photographers are the emotional first responders. I never want you to think that you 'must' wait to talk to a professional.

Debriefs can also be helpful when you're seeking independent childbirth education for a second or subsequent birth. When I used to teach the Hypnobirthing Australia course, the majority of couples I worked with were actually people who had experienced a previous traumatic birth. I talk more about the benefits of independent childbirth education in Chapter 15.

A DEBRIEF IS SELDOM A COMPLETE PROCESS

I think it's important to point out that you shouldn't expect everything to be fine just because you had a debrief. It might be that you have one and this is enough to get you where you want to be. If so, great, but working with trauma is a long-term process in my experience.

There are limits to what you can work through in one hour. A debrief isn't designed for behaviour change, goal setting and transformation. It's simply a brief container to hold your pain and validate it. Psychological debriefing was never intended to be a stand-alone intervention—rather it should be but one part of comprehensive, holistic care.

You also need to be mindful about filtering yourself. If you're only going to give someone the *Reader's Digest* version of your story, there are limits to your growth. Consider if you might be:
- trying to be a 'good' girl and not cause a fuss?
- trying not to get anyone into trouble

- holding yourself back in case you traumatise the person hearing your story
- assuming blame to yourself or your body without all the background information (e.g. energy levels and mood of staff that day, hospital policies on what counts as 'failure to progress', how many other people were birthing on the ward at the same time).

It should go without saying, but an effective debrief needs to be completely voluntary. The risks and benefits of participating need to be made clear. If you are being coerced into having a debrief, consider what the motive is. There is a history, at least with critical incident debriefing, where informed consent was not always sought. In fact, there is a history of organisations making people attend debriefs in an attempt to cover their arses. That is, trying to say 'You can't sue us! We gave you a debrief'.

You need to be fully aware that a debrief alone does not actually prevent you from developing post-traumatic stress disorder (PTSD). You might feel OK-ish around the time of the birth but then develop symptoms long after the event. I'm not saying this to scare you, just to be realistic that trauma doesn't follow a linear pattern.

If you decide to have a debrief, now you've got more information and questions to ask about how it's going to ensure you feel safe and validated.

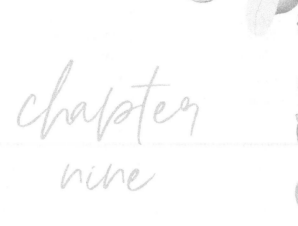

Phoenix Rising and Post-Traumatic Growth

Part of my passion and purpose is getting people to see, hear, feel, smell, and taste stress as a challenge instead of a threat. Trauma is our biggest teacher and a conduit for growth. Feeling good is your birthright. Part of you must have picked up this book because you want to feel better. Joy, fun and feeling good is part of that.

As I've explained before, a trauma response is your nervous system screaming 'Hey, I'm here! You're alive! Time to shake your meaning maker'. Post-traumatic growth is the antidote to post-traumatic stress. Broken is not a burden. It's a fucking blessing, a gift that is being handed to you. Even if it's not what you expected. Like that kid on YouTube who receives an avocado as a gift and is all 'avocado! … oh … thanks'.

We are becoming provocateurs of the pity party. Misery lit is one of the high rollers of the book world, and upwards of 90 per cent of the consumers of misery literature are women. You follow #birthtrauma and it's pretty much all shadow and darkness. Endless pity parties and emotional contagion. Venting and victim-identifying, which create hot air and reaction or, worse, inaction. Who is actually benefiting from this?

Inaction and pity as a response to trauma is not the legacy I want to leave, nor is it the content I create. We can do better than 'poor you'. The message is in the mess. My work is about finding the light, growth, strength and even joy. Hot air, if channelled well, could mean a balloon soaring high in the sky, with you shouting down below 'Look at me! I'm not fucking broken!'.

Post-traumatic growth is finding light in, not making light of, trauma. After a bushfire, trees regenerate and sprout new, lush foliage. Some ecosystems even thrive from fire. Australian gums hold their seeds locked in hard, wooden capsules. Fire causes the release of new seeds, and the ash beds that remain are perfect seed beds for new growth.

In kintsugi, precious broken objects are mended with gold so they are stronger and more beautiful. In martial arts, stress fractures hurt like hell, but they make the bones stronger.

Think for a minute about a horrific event that changes lives for generations—like the Holocaust. One mindset is to say 'It was so horrible, we can't and shouldn't enjoy anything because of what happened'. Another mindset is to say 'We must celebrate things and find joy *because* it happened'. Each of us has ancestral trauma. Let us not forget that women who were healers and helpers were once called witches. They were literally burnt before they had a chance to burn out.

You are the one your ancestors hoped for. Trauma is in your genetic lineage. It's turned on or off in your cells simply by what you choose to do with it. You can choose to do something meaningful with your misery.

In a nutshell, post-traumatic growth is transformation following trauma. You propel yourself forwards with strength and growth, in spite of what happened.

Resilience is different. Resilience is the personal attribute or ability to bounce back. With resilience you take a knock after trauma, and you feel low, but then your happiness levels go back to where they were.

With post-traumatic growth, on the other hand, you are knocked down, and you struggle to even lift your head up over the fog of misery. You never get back to that original state of happiness. But what's phenomenal is that you actually rise higher than you ever were. You shed your skin and then you're like the Hulk—stronger, happier and more powerful than before.

If resilience is the beautiful, but kind of expected, transformation of caterpillar into a butterfly, then post-traumatic growth is the phoenix rising. The 'well, that was fucking unexpected! How did you do that?'

Post-traumatic growth is not about your Pollyanna-ish 'Oh I'm so grateful this happened. Here's the deeper meaning' two seconds after the event happened. Growth is a process with seasons. It's about accepting what is (not what should have been and what might be) and thriving in spite of what happened. It's also accepting your own season of growth, that without the decay and desolation of winter, there wouldn't be spring.

Accepting trauma is not the same as liking it. And in case it isn't clear by now, let me say again that this has nothing to do with saying 'At least you've got a healthy baby'. A healthy baby is the baseline of what we should be aiming for, not the ceiling. I won't participate in selling birthing women the lie that basement-bargain-level outcomes are all we can hope for. Let's stop fixating on broken systems and broken birthing women, and instead break the glass ceiling.

All the time I hear of people saying things like 'this is just the way birth is', 'we need to toughen up', 'women are being special snowflakes' and so on. We expect people to be strong and resilient without giving them any real teachable skills in how to do this. We expect people to open up and share, without creating a safe container. Without training our birth workers in how to support women and themselves.

So how are you going to train yourself to see this shitty birth experience as a challenge instead of a threat? It's twofold. The dip-your-toe-in part is macro or global self-care. This is the bit people like. Taking care of your senses to stay healthy and feel better. This is your green smoothies. The walks on the beach, the massages, the bubble baths. These are the things you can photograph and pop on your Instagram feed. Awesome. Do all of that.

Most people will pick up a few strategies and stop there. They don't do the deep dive excavation work because it's super uncomfortable. Forget a bubble bath. This is diving into a bath of your own diarrhoea. The only real way to wade through is to learn to slay your own bullshit.

Personal growth and self-care. These are terms that sound lovely because calling it what it actually is—'deliberately making yourself uncomfortable, so uncomfortable you'd rather die than deal with your shit'—well, no-one wants to do that.

There is real value in sifting through your shit. I relish it! I'm like the laser-focused *kopi luwak* maker, and my clients are the civet from which the golden nuggets are extracted. *Kopi luwak* is the most expensive coffee in the world. It's extracted from the crap of a small cat-like creature. Don't you ever deny your own value.

There is a place for the future you to make less of the event of your birth. The what, the why, the where, the how and the when can fade into the background. Future you is going to be far more invested in these two questions:

1. What are you going to make it mean?
2. How have you become stronger, wiser and more unstoppable in spite of what happened to you?

THE BAMBOO TREE ANALOGY

These might not be questions you are ready for right now, but that's OK, we are simply planting the seed. One of my business coaches has often used the analogy of the bamboo tree. Like any plant, the bamboo tree requires nurturing. It needs water, fertile soil and sunshine. In its first year, there's zero sign that it's growing. In the second year, again, no growth and nothing happening above the soil. The third, the fourth, still nothing. Our patience is seriously tested and we begin to wonder why on earth we bothered planting this tree. Finally, in the fifth year, something different happens. We experience growth. Holy moly, your tree grows 2.5 metres in just six weeks!

Please don't cling to the five-year part. That is not the important part of the story. The important part is about realising that trauma work takes time, and often, just as you think nothing is happening, you'll hit growth. You might be washing your dishes or walking the dog and suddenly, things click into place. You're happier. You have more compassion and kindness towards yourself. You might dip and dive again, remember healing is not linear, but also remember that other annoying but useful saying: it's always darkest before the dawn.

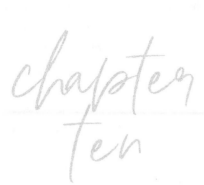

How to Find Holistic Support That Suits You and Your Family

You'll notice that this book is peppered with various holistic tools and approaches that I've found helpful. In this chapter, I want to walk you through a slightly more formal roadmap of treatment and support options. This might be useful if you're someone who prefers an evidence-based approach or you suspect you want specific guidance for a mental health problem. This is essentially what a psychologist or other mental healthcare professional might offer in their tool kit. My aim here is to cover some, but definitely not all, of what's available. Too much choice gets overwhelming in my experience.

Some people love researching loads of options, making pro and con lists and making an informed decision. Others just want two or three options and someone to quickly recommend something.

Here's some points to note before delving into to what's available:

1. There's no 'one thing' that will take it all away.
2. It's going to be uncomfortable. You need to expect that it will be. This is where growth happens.
3. You'll never be 'ready', but there are certainly things to think about setting up to help support you on starting your treatment/support (Are you in a safe, secure living situation? Is your general health OK? Can you make the financial investment in yourself? Do you have childcare? – not just for the appointments but for a buffer of time beforehand and after to process).
4. No matter which approach you choose, it's likely you might need to try a few approaches, and even practitioners, before you find the right fit. This is normal.
5. Everyone who experiences phenomenal growth, transformation and success has had help. You can't self-improve on your own. Oprah has help. Steve Jobs had support. if you want something you've never had, then you've got to do something you've never done before!

Remember what I said about big-T and little-T trauma? With PTSD, someone is highly unlikely to get through this experience without some expert help from someone who is a specialist. Be really careful about sharing your energy and your story with someone who has no real qualifications or experience in trauma work.

With PTSD, you can't just read a book, talk yourself out of it, or just go and spend money on soothing your senses. Well, you can, but it's unlikely going to lead to the long-term change that you want. Trauma work is uncomfortable. Period.

It's a nervous system response, so it's likely to need some specific input to restart, rewire and shift this stuck nervous system response. You definitely don't need to have a diagnosis of PTSD to get help. For a little-T trauma, someone might get through with a self-help book, and some other holistic support options.

Whether it's big-T trauma or little-T trauma, here are so many options available, yet so little research specific to birth trauma.

In this chapter I give an overview of:
Cognitive behaviour therapy (CBT) and other cognitive therapies
eye movement desensitisation and reprocessing
hypnotherapy
the rewind technique
somatic experiencing
the emotional freedom technique—'tapping'
animal-assisted therapy.

I also make mention of:
Chinese traditional medicine
holistic pelvic care
the practice of 'closing the bones'.

In the interests of not overwhelming you, this is an overview of the pros and cons of different approaches, and how to access them. I'm always trying to research and incorporate different cultures and practices, so this will probably change over time.

It takes a long time for an idea to become fully incorporated and accepted in medicine, and it's probably longer with mental health.

This is because a lot of what we are talking about is invisible, and measuring improvements relies on communication, rather than seeing physical results. This is why the medical model of 'find the problem, diagnose it, treat it and cure it' doesn't necessarily apply very well to trauma.

We also have people who still say things like 'it's all in your head'. I always have a laugh to myself when I hear this because, duh, your brain is responsible for every single part of your body! We dismiss invisible illnesses. It's also, arguably, much easier to get grants and funding for research where a financial backer can physically see the results. Just something to think about.

We have magnetic resonance imaging (MRI) research, and ways of looking inside people's brains to see results, but the average person isn't ever going to get an MRI or similar for mental health. Most things in psychology are diagnosed by observation. In part, that's because it's cheaper and more convenient.

People have different opinions about the best treatment approach for trauma. What suits one person may not suit someone else. What suited you at one time may not suit you later. If it helps and it's not harmful, I'm all for a holistic approach. Let's start with what the World Health Organization recommends for PTSD: cognitive therapies and eye movement desensitisation and reprocessing.

COGNITIVE THERAPIES

This is one of the main approaches I was trained in. If you are accessing counselling sessions through Medicare's Better Access scheme (or another scheme) then this is the main therapy approach that's used.

Within CBT there's a lot of thinking and talking about the traumatic event in detail. A large component of this approach is also writing—writing the event as it happened, in the past, then in the present.

In doing this, we look for what are called 'hot spots'. These are the particularly challenging thoughts, images, memories and automatic negative thoughts where the brain is stuck.

The goal is to work with thoughts and beliefs about the trauma so that distress is reduced. Cognitive approaches are based on the premise of replacing distressing thoughts with neutral or positive ones.

You may have heard of the Pavlov's dog experiment and the conditioning of a bodily reaction to a thought.[22] Pavlov was a Russian physiologist who won a Nobel prize for his work demonstrating the mind–body connection. In a nutshell, he starved some dogs, then showed them food and they would drool. He then began to ring a bell when he fed them so that eventually, just ringing the bell would make the dogs salivate.

Ringing a bell does not in and of itself cause a dog to drool. But the experimenter creates associations, and with repeated exposure conditions a reaction to an event or thought. A less cruel example of this is when you get a new puppy and you're taking them for a walk. Those first few times they have no idea what a lead is or what it represents (other than something to chew on). With repeated exposure, you might find that the mere act of you moving towards where the lead is kept and picking it up is enough to send your dog into an excited frenzy. The lead in itself is not exciting, but the dog now has paired the memories and feelings of going for a walk with this object.

As I've said before, your brain doesn't know the difference between what is real and what is imagined, hence exposure to images or thoughts works in the same way. Thinking about the traumatic event produces the same bodily reactions and the same fight-or-flight responses. So a psychologist or other mental health practitioner will actively evoke these responses, safely and carefully, and then work to change them. To teach the brain that the threat has passed and you are safe.

So again, cognitive approaches look at the thoughts that are creating the feelings and sensations. With repeated exposure to thoughts and memories about the trauma, we can retrain the brain. So, say one of the hot spots is the thought 'I'm going to die'. This was certainly one of mine from my first birth, and I experienced what's called a peritraumatic death imprint. It basically means that there was a point during the traumatic event where you really thought your life was in danger. People who experience this sometimes find that their brain gets 'stuck' on the feelings, thoughts and sensations that go with that snapshot. If you don't retrain your brain to know that the threat has passed (not just logically know but have your nervous system believe it), it can keep playing as a loop. With CBT we would carefully go over this distinct memory and pair it with a new thought: 'I'm going to get through this'. We'd also do some work around learning to shift out of fight-or-flight mode and teach your nervous system to no longer react to the thought. So, you learn to slow your breathing, release muscle tension and generally feel a lot calmer.

We do this multiple times, until those sensations like heart rate, sweating and shaking go down, and the person is able to think and talk about the event without the same emotion and distress attached to it.

If you listen to me talk about the traumatic parts of my births, I'm able to do so with less and less negative emotion every time I do it. That ability to speak about it with little emotion but still stay very much in the present and in my body—that's a practice effect. It still hurts. There are still some parts that are harder to live with than others, and I still cry, depending on the memory and the day.

You can then see how hard it can be when people have either shut off from the emotions of their trauma, or they've actually healed it, and then they have to go to court or appear in the media, and then people say Oh they don't seem upset about it—so maybe it didn't happen?'

Some people can describe their experiences with little to no emotion, but they are completely disconnected from their body and their surroundings when they do so. This is called dissociation, depersonalisation or derealisation. It's one of the brain's clever ways of protecting people from the anguish of the trauma. It can be protective and helpful, but it can become problematic if it's someone's primary coping strategy or it is impacting on their day-to-day life and relationships.

The goal with talking about your trauma isn't necessarily to feel positive, or to feel nothing, but with practice, it's definitely more tolerable and less scary to think about the birth than it used to be.

I still cry when I think about or talk about my births, but if I did that every single time I was trying to teach and translate skills, it wouldn't be very effective.

Cognitive Therapies: Pros

- It's evidence-based. There's longitudinal research (hundreds of thousands of articles over a long period of time) and it's supported by the WHO.
- It is also Medicare-rebate-supported.
- It's easy to find a practitioner with this training.
- The skills learned translate well into other areas of life.

In many cases, I would use this approach before the birth, if I know that someone is already terrified of birth. Teaching them coping statements and affirmations can definitely help to reduce the potential for a traumatic birth.

Cognitive Therapies: Cons

While CBT is potentially the best we have, it still doesn't cure all PTSD. The gold standard 'dose' of CBT for PTSD is 20-plus sessions, so roughly 12 months of work. When Medicare's Better Access scheme for mental health started in 2006, psychologists used to have 24 sessions to work with. The number of sessions offered through the Better Access scheme is currently less than the golden standard for treatment of PTSD. If you have PTSD, it's perhaps unlikely you'll see the results you're hoping for under the current scheme. This means you either have to fork out for the rest of the payments yourself or wait until a new calendar year to access further subsidised sessions. Not so useful if you want to start treatment in January.

Some people can also find CBT a bit 'blamey' if they read it as 'your thoughts are the problem'. I'm sometimes also wary about its use with sleep-deprived parents. Figuring out the nuances of your thoughts when you're putting your keys in the fridge and trying to remember if you fed the dog is hard work.

Even imaginal exposure (thinking about and talking about the event) is way too confronting for some people to deal with, so cognitive therapies are not great for people who don't remember much of their trauma, or who have trouble identifying their thoughts.

WHO CAN DELIVER CBT?

A psychologist, a social worker, some GPs, psychiatrists, psychiatric nurses and possibly counsellors and a few other professionals can do CBT. There are courses on CBT all over the internet now, but keep in mind that a weekend course is not going to be the same as a two-year master's degree and thousands of hours of experience.

EYE MOVEMENT DESENSITISATION AND REPROCESSING (EMDR)

In the 1980s, Francine Shapiro made the chance observation that eye movements could reduce the intensity of disturbing thoughts, under certain conditions. How it works is that the client identifies a specific problem as a focus for the treatment session. The client then calls to mind the disturbing issue or event—what was seen, felt, heard and so on. The therapist will then have the client initiate certain eye movements or other bilateral stimulation. Sometimes clients might hold some clickers in their hands, or they might use lights. Each practitioner will have their own techniques. These eye movements and other types of bilateral stimulation are used until the memory becomes less disturbing and is associated with a positive thought and belief about yourself.

EMDR: Pros

As I mentioned, EMDR is also supported by the WHO. It's an approach that's frequently used with war veterans. Most of the research is not specific to birth, but there are new articles coming out, and it's definitely something passionate researchers are working on.

EMDR can be useful if people aren't ready, aren't able to or don't want to talk about the trauma too much yet. People may start with EMDR and once they feel more confident, then they are able to start talk therapy. It usually integrates other therapies like CBT anyway, and Medicare has recently approved this modality for use under the Better Access scheme, meaning that you can sometimes get a rebate for sessions.

There is some evidence that EMDR is quicker than other therapies. About 77 to 99 per cent of people with PTSD were able to eliminate symptoms after three to seven sessions of EMDR. Remember that this research is not specific to birth trauma; it's just a guide.

EMDR: Cons

One of the drawbacks of EMDR is possibly the cost. While EMDR has recently been added to the list of modalities that Medicare will subsidise, not every mental health practitioner is trained in EMDR, nor do all of them offer a Medicare rebate.

You do need to find a specialist practitioner because as far as I know,

EMDR is not a standard part of psychologists' or psychiatrists' training. So only someone who has suitable qualifications (usually at least a master's degree in a relevant field) and then has completed specialist additional training can offer this service.

EMDR can be also be intense. So while it may be quicker, it's definitely not for the faint-hearted. You'd need really good support and not be attempting it in your lunch break.

There's really not much evidence about whether EMDR translates into online treatment yet, but I have heard of people delivering it this way, and after covid-19, I expect we will see more research soon.

ANIMAL-ASSISTED THERAPY

As you might guess, in animal-assisted therapy you get to work with horses, cats, dogs or other animals to work through trauma. PTSD often leaves people numb, yet animals can elicit positive emotions and warmth. Animals have also been demonstrated as social facilitators to connect people and build trust. The presence of an animal has also been linked to the release of oxytocin. It might be as simple as having a cat or a dog in your therapist's office, or some therapists may live outside the city and have several animals who frequent their property. Others will have a dedicated ranch or sanctuary where they primarily work outside with horses.

ANIMAL-ASSISTED THERAPY: PROS

This is potentially really good if you've got claustrophobia, but it can also be an adjunct to office-based therapy. Some therapists have a cat in their office or do additional training to have a therapy dog.

Animal-assisted therapy has great potential as a therapeutic tool when trust in people has been lost. And you can see the physical results. You can see the impact your emotions and body language have on an animal. The focus can also shift from being directly about you and your trauma to other skills when needed, such as learning to find confidence so that you can approach and work with a horse. So, it can be excellent for team building, stripping away the ego and levelling the playing field a bit.

ANIMAL-ASSISTED THERAPY: CONS

The downside is that there's still not a lot of rigorous research evidence. Again, it's not Medicare-supported, and there may be travel costs because you can't really do equine therapy in the CBD in your lunch break.

Typically, there's no standard protocol for how long it takes. There's also no current standard for assessing the welfare of the animals.

There are no rigorous guidelines about who can deliver this service. Some people are mental health practitioners, some are coaches. Someone might be very skilled with horses but not necessarily have the experience, training and skill to deal with severe trauma.

I've heard and read some amazing results, but again, it's still early days.

OTHER APPROACHES

This next section is an overview of some other approaches. Again, some will be a form of therapy or support you can seek training in from an expert, others will be techniques or tools you could try yourself. As always, be mindful that I am not giving medical or psychological advice here. Do your own research and take responsibility for your own healing. If you have PTSD, you'll likely need targeted support rather than trying to self-help your way through it.

EMOTIONAL FREEDOM TECHNIQUE

Emotional freedom technique (EFT), also called 'tapping', can be described as 'psychological acupressure'. People have mixed views about its efficacy, but it has become increasingly popular in the last few years. In many ways, it might be useful to think of this as a supportive tool rather than an entire therapeutic approach. You could seek out a practitioner solely for the purposes of being treated with EFT, but my way of thinking about it is that you would probably receive it for one session, in addition to other approaches.

I like EFT for a few reasons. One is that it uses 'teach a person to fish' principles. This is something you can teach yourself and use anytime, anywhere. It gives you something to 'do' other than work with your thoughts.

EFT combines coping statements, affirmations or positive self-talk with something physical. Often anxious people often need something productive to do with their hands! It's used for lots of different things like anxiety, depression, trauma and any thoughts or beliefs you want to shift.

Tapping is like acupuncture and acupressure (which is where you apply pressure without needles) is powerful. Acupressure is one of the strategies that got me through an induced birth without any other drugs, and through the birth of my 5 kg baby with stuck shoulders. I am a huge fan.

With EFT, you access different 'meridian' points, typically on the fleshy ('karate-chop') point of your hand, top of head, eyebrow, side of eyes, under eyes, under nose, above chin, collarbone, under arm and your wrist points.

You tap five to seven times gently on each point with your fingertips. (There are meridian energy points on the ends of your fingers, too!) Use your index and middle finger on your dominant hand or hands as you say each statement. You start by figuring out what you want to work on. For example, it might be feeling anxious when you think about your birth.

You'd start with giving a rating for how strongly you feel this from 0 to 10, with 0 being fine and 10 being 'I'm in full panic mode'. The goal is to work through rounds of tapping until the number reduces. The goal is not necessarily to get to zero! Maybe your natural 'rest' state is more like a 3 or 4.

You tap on each of the points for a few rounds, while focusing on the problem you have and accepting it. EFT works partially on the premise that negative feelings are hard to shift because we don't accept them. If we can accept them, they can be released.

There are loads of video demonstrations of EFT on YouTube, so you could essentially teach this to yourself. Remember what I said about diagnosable PTSD though: self-teaching is awesome, but I'm not suggesting you can shift full PTSD by yourself.

Again, this is something practical you can do while on the go. You can just use the karate-chop point if you're in a crowded waiting room, for example. We spent a great deal of our lives being told not to fidget, and yet doing something to move our bodies and move energy is actually incredibly helpful for the nervous system.

HYPNOTHERAPY

If you consider the importance of language and think about fears and the subconscious as it relates to birth, this approach just makes intuitive sense. It does for me. Now if we look at standard hypnotherapy for PTSD, there is a reasonably large meta-analysis (essentially a big review of available studies) from 2006 showing that hypnotherapy helps.[23] I go on about hypnobirthing a lot, because I've seen and experienced the results at first hand. Research on hypnobirthing is still really limited, but I've seen great results with clients who have previous birth trauma. And, of course, I've used it in both my births and I really found the combination of mindset, breathing, acupressure and other tools very helpful. However, you can still have a hypnobirth and experience birth trauma.

Hypnosis works by accessing the subconscious and rewriting negative thoughts, feelings and sensations with positive ones. Sometimes people have preconceived ideas of what 'hypnosis' means. Images of swinging pocket watches and being made to cluck like a chicken. Those are movie tropes, not facts. Even trained psychologists can be funny about the word 'hypnosis'. I've had old lecturers and colleagues say that it isn't a real thing, or that it's not evidence-based. I find this an interesting reaction because as I understand it, hypnosis is really not all that different from deep relaxation, guided imagery or meditation. Hypnosis is something you are guided through, it's not something done to you.

Hypnosis is one of the oldest 'mind' techniques we have and was used to help patients through surgery before anaesthesia was invented. Hypnotherapy can be awesome for pain, both anticipatory pain, when someone fears the pain of childbirth and maybe can't use pharmacological pain relief, and also ongoing pain from birth, work or other injuries.

Who Can Deliver Hypnotherapy?

There are specific qualifications for hypnotherapists, though regulations about doing hypnosis are not particularly tight. So you want to check someone's qualifications and experience, not just accept any random person who says they do hypnosis. Not every mental health practitioner will be trained in hypnotherapy and it's not covered by Medicare.

REWIND TECHNIQUE

I'm hearing more and more about this technique for birth trauma, but again, not a lot of empirical evidence just yet. Rewind uses graduated imaginal exposure. It was first used for phobias and then adapted for treatment for PTSD. In brief, it gets you to imagine your trauma and to learn techniques to distance yourself from the event and the emotions of it.

People like rewind technique because it has a relatively short turnaround for results, and you don't necessarily need to go into loads of detail about your trauma. Again, it's a specialised technique, so someone would need to have completed the training.

SOMATIC EXPERIENCING

This one excites me because there's new research coming out all the time. It's based on Peter Levine's work and incorporates a lot of ancient wisdom with modern treatment principles. So, it connects the mind and body together in its approach, in which trauma is viewed as an incomplete defensive reaction.

The goal is to release the traumatic activation through an increased tolerance of bodily sensations and related emotions, allowing discharge. So there really is a big emphasis on understanding it and regulating the nervous system.

Most trials are limited to combat research, natural disasters and terrorism, but there are perinatal professionals who offer somatic experiencing. Only people with a relevant base qualification like psychology or counselling can deliver this technique. They then need to complete recognised somatic experiencing training, which takes about two years.

ALTERNATIVE TREATMENTS

In this section I want to draw your attention to some holistic support options that may help. I want to acknowledge that I'm a privileged white woman who was trained in techniques mostly developed by white men and tested on other white people. Just because something is researched and funded, doesn't mean it's gospel.

For example, Chinese traditional medicine has been around much longer than Western approaches. In Australia, it's endorsed and often covered by private health insurance, so it's an alternative to or complement to Western medicine.

Trauma is obviously linked to the adrenal system and the kidneys among other things, so it really helps balance the body and emotions. Chinese medicine can help you get pregnant, help with nausea or pain, natural induction, turn breech or posterior babies and generally keep things in balance. A Chinese medicine practitioner can also help with postpartum depletion, stress and improved wellbeing through improved energy flow.

Then there's also holistic pelvic care, which was developed by Tami Lynn Kent using physical and energetic tools to address chronic tension and pelvic imbalances. Tami has worked with over 10,000 women and her TED talk is a good one to watch. The techniques are designed to address the tension and pelvic congestion to enhance overall pelvic, vaginal health and a general sense of wellbeing. I do know of at least one holistic GP in Australia who does this work (Dr Danielle Arabena).

And lastly for this section, let's briefly look at 'closing the bones'. This is a traditional South American practice, although it's used in other cultures too. It acknowledges that the hips widen from pregnancy and birth, and it uses a series of wrappings to physically close the pelvis. It also calls the person's spirit back into their body and some people find it emotionally helps them to close the chapter of difficult birth.

Before we close this chapter, I want to draw your attention to some important points about treatment for trauma.

TREATMENT ISSUES

As you would expect, there is no one single treatment that serves all people with trauma. More than 40 per cent of people with PTSD don't respond to first-line treatment,[24] and this is something that's not made clear nearly often enough. The risk of reactive feelings of shame and failure when a treatment doesn't work is high, so I really feel we need to be teaching people not to blame themselves if relief isn't instant. They may need to try a few things.

In psychology, we have something called the dodo hypothesis (or dodo verdict or conjecture) that you could do any validated psychotherapy and achieve similar results. It's a controversial topic, but one well worth considering. Now, here are some things I want you to consider when looking for support.

THINGS TO NOTE WHEN SEEKING SUPPORT

As you might have figured out by now, birth trauma is not something that even really highly trained people necessarily know about. Again, it's a gap in training. There are GPs, psychologists and psychiatrists who are savvy and interested in perinatal work. But if it's a case of who you can get in to see right now, then you might have to be prepared to some educating and prompting about what you need. This is actually a huge burden, which is why doulas and other advocates have such a huge role to play.

Birth is still left off so many of the infographics about PTSD. Perinatal mental health isn't specifically covered in most training in psychology, social work or counselling. It's an extra area of interest, training and expertise, so where possible you want to find someone who at least has some experience and understanding of the nuances of the perinatal period.

One good question to ask might be: 'How would you know if what I'm experiencing is postnatal depression/anxiety or PTSD?'. A common thing I've seen over my years of practice is women getting a diagnosis of postnatal depression, taking antidepressants and then not improving.

If the professional is not looking for trauma as a possibility, they won't see it in their assessment of you. The rule of thumb is that people who are anxious or depressed are not stuck in a perpetual loop of panic specifically about the birth and experiences immediately afterwards. Their experiences are more general. Maybe there's trauma *and* anxiety, or PTSD, or something else. The professional should look at all possibilities and what's happening for the individual in front of them. I really think we need so much more time to get to know people and what's going on in the different areas of their life.

I also think it's good to ask, 'How do you differentiate sleep deprivation, poor eating, hormonal shifts and other typical postpartum experiences from a mental health problem?'

Does the person you're asking seem humble, willing to see you as an individual and say 'I don't know' if they don't know?

Do they seem rigid or inflexible, for example saying CBT is the only thing that will work for you? Do they baulk at the idea of trying alternative approaches?

Do they understand and appreciate your culture and preferences? An Indigenous woman who has experienced obstetric violence and/or poor care from a team of white birth professionals probably doesn't want to see a nice white lady for therapy. In fact, the research tells us that having access to a health professional who has the same ethnicity, religion, cultural background to yourself means better outcomes.[25] A recent study in the US found that newborn black babies are three times more likely than white babies to die in the hospital when their care providers are white.[26] I have seen some truly racist and uninformed hospital guidelines written about how to care for Black, Asian, Indigenous and Hispanic patients. You have a right to seek another healthcare provider if the one in front of you isn't meeting your needs.

These are just a few things to keep in mind, so that you're more likely to get specialised help.

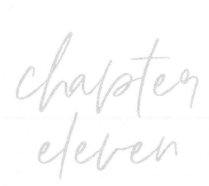

chapter
eleven

Tried Getting Support and It's Not Working? Problem Solving

In the last chapter I mentioned that you might need to try a few different approaches and even a few different practitioners before you find the right fit. This is normal. It's a pain in the arse, but it's all too common with trauma and not talked about nearly enough, in my view.

Let's say you've taken that first step and have reached out for support and it's feeling like it's not helping or you're not seeing the results you want. I don't want this to be read as a 'the problem is you' or 'your therapist sucks' attack. It's super difficult not to take things personally, because trauma and birth are so personal. If you're feeling stuck, see if you can pull back, get a second opinion from someone you trust and see if any of the common scenarios below ring true. It's not about blaming and pointing fingers; this is about finding solutions.

Here are seven of the most common stumbling blocks.

1. THE CONTAINER THAT NEEDS TO HOLD YOU HAS HOLES

While there is no perfect time to start 'the work', there are a few basic but important conditions that need to be met first. You can Google Maslow's hierarchy of needs. Even I forgot about this basic requirement before starting my own coaching for exhaustion. In a nutshell, there are basic necessities that humans require to be met before they can manage any higher-level activities. Sleep, food, safe shelter, warmth and so on. You simply can't do a whole lot of growth if you're just surviving or in active crisis mode. It's something that can't be overlooked, but often is.

I think often about when I used to work with the homeless. All the time family and friends would say 'wow, that must be so rewarding, you're helping so much'. Yes and no. All I could really do is put out spot fires, and help people manage their pain and conflicts in the short term. You can't go home and practise mindfulness if you don't know where you're even going to sleep that night. Or if you're hungry or haven't showered and are distracted by all your thoughts and feelings of shame about how your therapist must be judging you because you stink. You can't retain information about coping strategies if all you can think about is whether your stuff is going to get stolen or you're going to get bashed or arrested. Many of our clients were still actively using drugs to cope, and so that limited what we can expect for problem-solving and memory.

Here's an analogy using the physical body. The pre-game work hasn't been done. You haven't stretched, slept, eaten or hydrated before trying to run a marathon. You haven't planned ahead—you

don't know when your next snack or drink of water will be, you haven't broken in your running shoes (or put tape on your nipples to prevent chafing—apparently that's a thing!), and hell, you don't even really know where you're going.

For therapy to 'work' you first need to be managing to be human. If you don't sleep enough, you're going to look like you're in a mental health crisis anyway. If cameras in my house were to capture me on those days where I've barely had two hours of sleep, I would look like I'm in acute crisis mode—endless tears, irritability, startling easily, crashing into things, being totally out of my body and maybe even hallucinating a little. If I headed to a mental health practitioner in that state, they'd diagnose me with a mental illness for sure (unless they knew me and took the time and care to actually look at me like a whole person).

Maybe you've got some messy corners in your life and you're trying to skip ahead to the outcome and fast-track your way to growth without attending to the boring shit like sleep and diet. I know I have been in that space before.

There's no checklist of perfect things to check off before you start. Remember that you'll never be ready, but there is a huge difference between being in acute crisis and surviving and being OK enough to allow yourself to believe you are safe and nourished and use your brain.

2. THINKING THAT THE 50-MINUTE APPOINTMENT IS THE WORK
I've seen it time and time and time again. Thinking that booking

the therapy and turning up to the appointment is the work. The snarky offender on a community corrections order who is given an order to 'do anger management' or go to jail. So literally all they do is turn up, say they are fine, they couldn't possibly have any issues to work on, and ask if they can just read a magazine to pass the time. They keep reiterating that the magistrate said they just had to attend, not participate, just show up. Oh yes, that has happened to me many times!

It's also happened with parents of school-aged children who have thrown their black Amex at me across the desk and said that little Johnny or Janie is very busy. They don't have time to do work outside of these sessions. They ask what is so unreasonable about asking me to see their five-year-old at six o'clock at night. They have violin and maths club and pony club to get to, and they are very busy too. They look at their child's drawing that they did in session and ask 'is that all you did?'. They have no understanding of rapport-building or trust or the importance of play and expect me to 'fix' the problem in three sessions.

What you do in those 50 or so minutes of your psychology or other appointment is maybe not even a quarter of the work. The person doing 95 per cent of the work should be you—not your therapist.

It's not just about booking a 50-minute appointment, it's about giving yourself a buffer. What are you doing before the appointment? What are you going to do straight afterwards? Expecting to do therapy for trauma in your lunch break and then head back to work or whiz off to pick up the kids and hope to be present with them will slow your progress.

If your partner is not on board with you investing in yourself then that will slow your progress. If you haven't got adequate child support, healthy foods that are ready to be thawed from the freezer or delivered, then that will slow your progress. Many people who begin any kind of trauma work start to get sick, either as a physical manifestation of things moving and shifting, or as a self-handicapping strategy (easier to get permission for the flu than for your mental health?).

Growth and healing are not convenient. Think about any major challenge in your life. Was it conveniently timed? Did you get pregnant at the 'perfect' time, birth at the 'perfect' time? Is this a long-term goal you're investing in and prioritising or is healing something you're hoping to do on the side?

It's not about setting a perfect plan in place! Micromanaging your healing won't work either, but allow space and nourishment for yourself wherever possible in all senses of those words.

3. YOUR THERAPIST (OR POSSIBLY THE SERVICE) ISN'T THE RIGHT FIT

Both the process and content have to be in alignment. They must have the right content (they have the tools, knowledge and skills to help you) *and* the process. This is all the nonverbal stuff: how you feel in their presence? Do you even like them? Do you feel like they think they are better than you? Do they see you as whole and the best version of you or only another 'broken' human? Do they even like babies? I'm serious. Some people are great at the mental health part but are not able to be flexible if the babysitter cancels, or can't understand why you can't turn your phone off.

The therapeutic relationship (the process) is so important. Possibly even more important than what approach you choose (the content). This is the person who you are allowing to know your soul—better and deeper than any lover, friend or family member.

I have always said to clients: mental health is not like other forms of health appointments. You can, in theory, choose a dentist who does great work, charges the right price, but actually is a bit of a prick. But you have to like your therapist. You have to feel they see you, are here for you and see it as an honour just to get to work with you.

I grew up in a small town where choice for healthcare providers was limited. Further, I was socialised to believe that healthcare providers were the experts, so it shouldn't matter so much if you didn't like them.

My parents are Scottish, raised in postwar poverty. My mother will return a tough piece of beef in a heartbeat, but would she complain about an arrogant, patronising healthcare practitioner? Nope. Not a chance. Maybe if they caused physical harm, but it's better not to make a fuss or have the inconvenience of changing.

That said, do give practitioners a chance. First impressions are not always fair. Remember how much we like to put other people's flaws down to character but expect others to see that it's situational when it comes to ourselves? Like the idiot who is tailgating and speeding past you on the road? An incompetent driver? An impulsive, impatient person? Maybe. Or maybe it's someone who has a partner in active labour, or a mum who is on her last breaths in a nursing home, or a child who has been injured at school. How would you know?

If you're not feeling treasured, fully attended to and supported after a couple of sessions it might be time to move on. It's not always personal. Trauma, as I've mentioned before, is so influenced by the subconscious. It might be that the person you've booked with has the same name as a teacher who was horrid to you in school. You may not like their perfume. They might be too old and you're experiencing transference issues (e.g. a man with a certain tone of voice and mannerisms is just always going to make you feel 15 years old and in trouble even though you logically know the person in front of you is not your dad).

You might think their taste in artwork and furnishings is hideous and thus subconsciously (or consciously) think 'if I don't trust their judgement in X then I can't trust it at all'. Being picky is OK. Being picky to use this an avoidance strategy or to stay in your 'I'm broken and no-one can help me' story is something else. Check in with that.

- There are other reasons why the fit might not be right: The practitioner just doesn't know enough about the postpartum period. Or they don't have the right support themselves from a mentor to guide them in what they need to best support you.
- The practitioner is pregnant, or trying to get pregnant, and this impacts her ability to fully attend to you. It shouldn't make a difference, but actually it does. On rare occasions it has happened that a client has been booked in to see me when (a) she didn't know I was pregnant and (b) neither I or reception knew that she

was coming for infertility or pregnancy loss or another issue where sitting across from a pregnant therapist would add an extra layer of pain for her.

- The practitioner has too many other clients on their books and is not fully able to give you the time and energy you need.

4. YOU'D RATHER STAY IN YOUR VICTIM STORY, SO YOU SELF-SABOTAGE

You're not going to like what I have to say here, but I feel that if you're having a strong reaction to this sentence above, you'll already know that this is your truth.

The brain likes things that are familiar. Your wounded self wants to keep you in your story to keep you safe and small. It's part of the reason why some people stay in domestic violence situations. It's one reason why people stay addicted to drugs. It's a huge part of why so many abused and neglected children almost always feel 'obligated' to their parents and want to go back to their care rather than live in foster care.

If you've been living in the 'I'm broken', 'I'm too much', 'I'm too traumatised' victim story for a while now, part of you may be afraid to discover who you are without that story. It's OK to acknowledge that maybe a part of your ego likes the concern and care that you receive from others because you are always struggling. It might well be that you've grown up in environments where the only way to receive love and attention is to be broken somehow. Or that the only way to be special and interesting is through your traumas. Those are stories, not reality.

I've met plenty of people who say that therapy doesn't work. That they've tried everything. And absolutely, sometimes that's true. But if you want something you've never had before then you need to do something different from everything you've ever done. Many of the people who have sat across from me and given me some spiel about how this won't work, how it 'never works', are correct. Whether you think you can or you can't, both are true. Much easier to blame everyone else for not being able to help you when you've actually never had any intention of being helped.

5. YOU'RE ONLY WINDOW SHOPPING FOR TREATMENT, YOU'RE NOT ALL IN

Window shopping is a normal part of any behaviour change. In psychology, we talk about how clients will circle in and out of different stages of change: pre-contemplative (not really interested), contemplative (window shopping, as I call it), action phase (ready to make change), maintenance (making the changes work consistently) and then sometimes relapse (I was doing all the things and then I fucked up).

You've already done this in some area of your life, whether it's committing to a new behaviour or quitting an old one. In drug rehab work we go around and around and around with these states, sometimes for decades.

If you suspect you're not all in, then do a pro and con list. This works for any behaviour. I've used it with ice addicts, repeat offenders, adolescents engaging in self-harm, people with eating disorders and people who are stuck in the idea that they can't get better or give up the thing.

A huge part of my career is convincing people to do things they don't want to do. Selling them things they don't want to buy and making changes they never ever think are possible.

When you're trying to convince someone to do something they don't want to do—let's use the example of 'just say no' to teens using drugs—a huge part of the missing picture is acknowledging the pros and the cons. Think about it. People wouldn't inject heroin if there was nothing positive about it. People stick to behaviours when there's a benefit even if it seems a bit warped.

Look at people in domestic violence situations. If it were as simple as 'just leave', it wouldn't be an issue. Please do not mistake this for me saying there are positives to staying in domestic violence. What I'm saying is that when you're so deep in discomfort and your nervous system and brain are used to it, you're so deep in survival mode that it can be hard to make new decisions. The person living with an abuser is thinking 'My kids have a bed, and their toys are here', 'What am I going to do with our pets?', 'I don't want to leave our house'.

Do your honest pro-and-con list. What are the beneficial reasons to not get help, stay stuck and not be all in? Be honest. Maybe, you would prefer that holiday to Bali rather than pay for therapy, so a positive is that you get to save money (in the short term). Maybe you really do believe that you need to work all this out for yourself and so the perceived benefit is the 'I'll show you' response at not needing anyone's help?

If you've been in treatment or multiple treatments for some time and you've never had this pro-and-con conversation with your care provider, now might be the time to look at it.

6. YOU'VE SET (OR BEEN SOLD) UNREALISTIC EXPECTATIONS

In Australia, at the time of writing, Medicare will subsidise some sessions with a psychologist or other eligible mental healthcare practitioner if you have a referral (and a diagnosis) from your GP. It sounds great, and I'm aware that in most countries, government-funded healthcare of any sort is unheard of. However, this means that sometimes people are inadvertently sold the idea that healing can be complete in the number of sessions that are rebated. The 'gold standard' for CBT for PTSD is close to a year's worth of sessions. The Better Access scheme was never intended to be used for chronic issues. I've spent many a mentoring session with a new psychologist trying to teach them what they can do for a client with PTSD in 10 or so sessions. It's frustrating and anxiety-provoking and can lead to both client and therapist feeling the experience was just carrot-dangling at best. Getting halfway through your progress only to have to find the money to keep going to wait until a new calendar year ticks over so you can access another few sessions is not a system that works very well.

If you're experiencing a little-T trauma, then maybe a few sessions of CBT will give you the support you need, but for PTSD it's unlikely to have dramatic results.

Clients always want to know how long treatment will take, and everyone has a different reaction. Some see it as a race, something to get in and out of as soon as possible. I've seen clients on a community corrections order from a magistrate try to book multiple sessions with me in a week so that they can tick a box. Growth is not linear. You can't plan too much.

Beware of anything that seems like a quick fix, particularly if it's something with zero research evidence support. Trauma is a very popular mental health issue at the moment. Psychology goes through fads, just like everything else, and there are plenty of people looking to make a buck by selling the proverbial snake oil. Talk to anyone who has navigated trauma—it's hard work. It takes time. It takes investing in yourself.

Approaches like Rewind or eye movement desensitisation and reprocessing (EMDR) may take fewer sessions, but usually the work is more intense. If you want quicker results and you can access these approaches, then go for it, but be discerning. The medical model of 'find, diagnose, treat and cure' doesn't fit well with trauma. We can't simply scan your brain, find the trauma, remove it and send you on your way.

7. TALKING ISN'T ENOUGH, OR YOU HAVEN'T YET BUILT THE EMOTIONAL RESERVES TO BE ABLE TO COMMIT TO TALK THERAPY

Talking about your trauma is possibly one of the most difficult parts of navigating that experience. If you're diving straight in, you will need skills in how to slow down your breath and heart rate, pause and come back to the present, and other embodiment techniques. Without such skills you will find talking about your trauma even harder. In my view, talking about trauma is a like a muscle that needs to be built up. Like when you're surfing, you need to know that it's important to fall. Falling over and over is uncomfortable but it allows your brain to figure out how to stop you from falling. Learning how to fall—how to work with your nervous system when things start getting intense—is a pretty important step. Talking to your care provider about what happened (if you can even access it) comes later. Practitioners all work differently, and this is just my view.

For many people, talking about the 'what' can take multiple attempts. Doing some work on processing the trauma without going into detail about what happened (like with EMDR or Rewind) can be useful before you start talk therapy. Oher people really want to share the story. Our brains are wired for storytelling and working things out as we put them into a narrative. I have to admit that hearing people's stories is probably one of my favourite parts of my work. Receiving and holding space for people's stories is just part of my DNA.

Some days you'll plan to talk about the trauma and then it just doesn't happen. You're distracted by something else in your life, you need to cancel, a new stressor has come up or you have a really crappy night with the kids and just don't have the reserves to push too hard that day. Expect detours and setbacks because that is just human experience.

Of course, there are other variables not mentioned here. This is not an exhaustive list by any means, just a starting point.

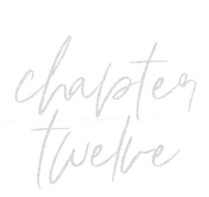

Breastfeeding Trauma

Breastfeeding can trigger huge feelings of failure, shame, self-doubt, guilt and a crushing sense of loss of bodily autonomy. Whatever your personal story and belief system, it is not under judgement or attack here. My discussion of my experiences and opinions on what was right for me is in no way intended to take away from your experience. Remember the adage 'her success is not your failure'.

I highly recommend you listen to my podcast episode with Amberley Harris. Amberley was my breastfeeding consultant for my second baby, and what she doesn't know about boobs and babies isn't worth knowing. We unpack all the predisposing, perpetuating, precipitating and protective factors around my breastfeeding experiences. I've also been interviewed on the Australian breastfeeding podcast with Susie Prout.

Breastfeeding as a traumatic experience is often overlooked. It can represent a continuation of traumatic birth, come up as a new trauma in and of itself, or trigger previous abuse or unpleasant associations and memories with our own bodies.

With my first baby I really struggled. Hand on heart, I don't think I've ever felt so low in my life as I did in those four weeks of attempting to breastfeed Stella. Nothing has made me feel more disappointed, isolated and like a total failure as a human than that experience. If that has been even remotely like your experience, know that I'm here empathising with you. From the get-go, I already had the anticipation that breastfeeding probably wasn't going to work. That one mindset block led to a cascade of self-sabotage and hindsight bias. The best way that I know how to unpack it is with a technique that's used in counselling, called the 'four Ps analysis'. You can find a full summary on my website, but here's an overview:

PREDISPOSING (THE 'WHY ME?')
I had pre-existing expectations that breastfeeding would be difficult due to a range of reasons.

The first was anatomy ('flat nipples'). But really, if we look carefully at this, it was not so much my anatomy but the way that language around my anatomy was used. When my obstetrician examined me she said words to the effect of 'you might struggle to get a baby to latch'. She was optimistic and outlined support and things to try, but really all I heard was 'you're flawed and it will be difficult or not work'. That's not what she said, of course, but this is what I made it mean.

When Stella was born and I was trying to feed her, a midwife said to me 'oh you can't help the way you're born'. This again had the effect of giving an exhausted, non-confident mother the message that she was flawed, broken or incapable. I'd just come out of surgery. I'd just had two blood transfusions. This wasn't helpful to hear.

Later on, with my second baby, Amberley said to me 'Well, actually your baby only knows *your* nipples. She doesn't know any different and you'll work it out'. That was the confident reassurance I needed. Personally, I'd rather have someone who was overconfident in my ability, and have me prove them wrong, than have them start at a point of zero or low confidence in me so that I had to prove them right.

I also had a family history of 'not being able to' breastfeed. I'm not sure why exactly. I think a lot of us have this messaging in our family history. My mum says her milk 'just didn't come in'. She had a physiological birth, two hours total and no drugs. She hadn't been able to feed my older brother either. It's worth noting that in the early 1980s, it was becoming popular for formula companies to market to exhausted parents and overworked midwives by having product available. It must have seemed like a win–win.

My mother clearly had milk come in at some point, because she was prescribed drugs to 'dry up' any milk that did come in. She was then apparently shamed by her midwife, who kept pointing out how lucky she was to have these drugs because they were very expensive. My mum has also shared her feelings of feeling like a failure, when she had done everything right (that is, she didn't smoke or drink and she ate well). Even now, as a woman in her

70s, she'll say 'It wasn't fair! The woman next to me was guzzling Coke and sucking down fag after fag and her milk was flowing'.

Stella was never properly assessed for tongue-tie. Retrospectively, I don't know if this is something Stella may have experienced, but I wonder. I also know there are different views on whether tongue-ties are a variation of normal anatomy or something that needs to be surgically altered. What I do know is that lots of parents say this is something that wasn't assessed or considered in their breastfeeding difficulties.

Another predisposing factor was in my language. I'd said I would try to breastfeed, instead of saying 'I'll do this, and if it's hard I'll get help'. I was telling my subconscious that I wasn't 100 per cent sure I could do it. In hypnobirthing classes I used to teach students that it was better to focus on the outcome you did want and use that language, for example 'I will have X type of birth' or 'I will breastfeed'. If, in the event that circumstances are different, who cares? The person who would dare say to a new parent 'Oh, but you said you were going to ...' is not a friend worth having.

PRECIPITATING ('WHY NOW?')

With Stella I had a diagnosis of gestational diabetes. I didn't require medication, but from around 28 weeks of pregnancy I was pricking my finger and testing my blood five times a day. It never once spiked after the initial high reading from the glucose tolerance test. I have a lot of opinions about how gestational diabetes is assessed and managed cross-culturally. I have a lot of opinions about how birthing women with *any* health diagnosis in pregnancy are sometimes treated. I know how much guilt and shame I felt, and at times undertones of being treated like a naughty child. And that's from my highly privileged experience as a white, middle-class, cisgendered woman. I cannot fathom how it feels when you are already vulnerable, scared and suspicious of healthcare and are legitimately treated like an idiot. When black women are blamed for having hypertension instead of dismantling the trillion-dollar food industry that has caused the hypertension. I have a lot of strong opinions about health, poverty and the food industry. I also think this is a good point to acknowledge that generations of white babies were fed from black women who were forced to let their own babies perish. The history of wet-nursing in enslaved people is worth researching. The history of huge companies marketing low-cost, highly addictive unhealthy food to families in poverty is worth researching.

Going back to the birth of Stella, my diagnosis of gestational diabetes led to an induction, a very speedy delivery, and a baby with low blood sugar. Now did she have low blood sugar from my diabetes or because she was shocked after being expelled from my body with too much synthetic oxytocin too soon? I don't know. Either way, I had a large internal tear and a postpartum haemorrhage where I lost close to two litres of blood. I kept myself as calm as I could for as long as I could, but my body knew something wasn't right. I went into fight-or-flight panic mode and was experiencing 10/10 pain. I had a horrific attempted vaginal exam. I couldn't be examined, I was in so much pain. I went for emergency surgery genuinely thinking I might die. I then had two blood transfusions. By the time it was 7 p.m. I had not eaten anything since 5 a.m. except half a cheese sandwich. When the cheeseburger and chocolate mud cake I'd so been looking forward to for my first meal after the birth arrived, I was told I wasn't well enough to eat it. So, I was given a bullshit white bread and ham sandwich and watched as my husband ate my dinner looking so guilty. Is it any wonder that my body went 'hell no' to producing breastmilk? I still wanted to attempt it. Breastfeeding was important to me, but I wish someone had bloody told me about antenatal expressing beforehand (more on that later).

The first feed felt very rushed. I wasn't ready, she wasn't ready and I went into people-pleasing mode. My baby was shoved onto me with constant helpful reminders that she had low blood sugar and was hungry. I even think someone helpfully warned me that she could have a seizure if I didn't feed her soon.

There was no beautiful breast crawl, or chance for her to find her own way. I really don't even remember if we got a full golden hour of skin-on-skin time. All I remember was pain, bruises and blood blisters from the first feed and a baby with scrunched hands who kept turning her head away. She wasn't interested in eating and she was being forced. Even now, as a four-year-old, if Stella does not want to eat, she has a big emotional reaction. I'm mindful to give her the choice of when and how much she eats.

PERPETUATING ('WHY DOES IT CONTINUE?')
My milk was slow to come in after the haemorrhage and surgery, so the difficulties continued. I found the change of shift times really difficult. Just as I'd got to know someone and bonded with them, and let them 'milk' by boobs while I lay there utterly shattered, it was time for them to leave again and I'd have to start over with someone new.

I also witnessed arguments and bickering between staff about whether to I should choose formula or keep expressing colostrum. People discussed my 'ability' to breastfeed in front of me like I was livestock.

One of the midwives who saw me a few times during the nights was someone I didn't like at all. She may have been a nice person, but she sucked as a midwife. She was rude, patronising and inattentive. And yet I just kept letting her touch me. Because I was exhausted. Because I wanted it to be over with. Because I wanted to be a 'good girl' and not make a fuss. When I read this, I'm using the same language that victims of abuse use. If this is coming up for you right now, take a breath. Put the book down for a second and come back into your body—where are you, what year is it? Remember that the trauma is not happening right now and that you are safe.

In what other universe would I normally allow someone to treat me like this? To handle my naked body roughly, say stupid, patronising things and generally make me feel like shit? And yet birthing women are so vulnerable. We cannot expect them to have to fight for their own basic rights when they are in survival mode, when really their only job should be to have peace and get to know their baby. This midwife kept asking what meds I was on, what my dose was supposed to be and so on. How the fuck was I supposed to know that? I later found out she'd crossed off one of the anti-inflammatory medications on my chart, saying I couldn't have it due to interaction effects. This turned out to not be true at all and it was only on the final day that a new midwife looked at my chart and went 'that's not right'.

It pissed me off that she didn't bother to learn Stella's name even though it was written up on a whiteboard. She kept assuming that my baby was a boy because she was wearing grey and she was bald (wtf???). Every single visit, she kept saying my baby was hungry and if I hadn't learned to breastfeed by now, I wouldn't be able to breastfeed ever. The final nail in the coffin was her saying it wasn't fair for me to 'let it go hungry' (yes, calling my baby an 'it'). Woulda coulda shoulda. I should have learned her name and complained formally. But I was too tired and felt broken and just wanted to go home. So I filled out the feedback card and let rip about how unprofessional their night staff were. I'd learned the names of the midwives who were great and was sure to mention them by name.

The round-the-clock hand-expressing by different people often felt like assault. Being milked by a stranger making small talk about the weather (or worse, trying to talk to me about work 'so, why do you think people take drugs then, eh?') was weird. I was discharged from the hospital with the tick of approval that I was breastfeeding. In truth, I'd already outstayed my welcome with six nights in hospital, and I still had no idea what I was doing. I was super thankful that I'd already purchased a really high-quality pump. I can't imagine having to wander around Baby Bunting bleary-eyed, with boobs leaking, and looking for a pump. It was bad enough when my husband and I went to buy a new microwave oven when I was 39 weeks pregnant. I was so sick of being asked about when I was due that I told a lady it was just a big lunch. She looked at me like I was being so rude. I didn't care.

In the course of four weeks, I'd seen three lactation consultants and been given three different, completely inconsistent opinions. The environment of the breastfeeding clinic was also not ideal—

flickering fluorescent lights, vinyl chairs that were cold and made farty noises, and no windows. I forgot about 80 per cent of what I was taught. In contrast, my second breastfeeding attempt with Lily (which I'll discuss later), being in my own home with my husband remembering everything, was completely different.

With Stella, I couldn't find a lactation consultant who would come to our home so close to Christmas. I made a few phone calls and then gave up. I simply didn't have the stamina to keep trying.

Because I had no idea what I was doing, and had no-one to help me, I kept re-injuring my nipples—lipstick nipple, vasospasm, constant bleeding and cracking. I kept putting bras and shirts on to protect my modesty in front of visitors and this resulted in me ripping the skin off anytime I opened my bra. I told people not to visit, because I was so damn uncomfortable all the time and didn't want to subject them to my bleeding cracked nipples. I was also deeply embarrassed and ashamed. In hindsight, my sister-in-law who was visiting from the USA probably would have helped me. She offered many times, but I just couldn't let her in. At the time I had deep, trauma wounds from school. Women in the past had let me down terribly. I'd been bullied, singled out and physically assaulted by girls at school. I had a few close female friends, but they were all back in Tasmania and I was in Melbourne. Being weak in front of other women was not an option for me at that time.

Around week three, I was just too sore, anxious and angry about trying to re-attach Stella, so I just stuck to pumping to give my boobs a break. I was on the edge of becoming depressed so I decided I'd just pump. I had so much milk that had to come out somehow anyway, so I just kept going. In hindsight, I probably could have attempted to feed Stella from the breast again once they'd healed. However, I still had no direct support and the idea simply turned my stomach. I actually damaged one of my toes one day by digging it into the ground so hard when we were attempting to latch.

PROTECTIVE ('WHAT HELPS?')

As I've mentioned, I had no difficulties with expressing. I was prepared with my hospital-grade pump, and it didn't seem to take that long to fill a bottle. That is absolutely not the case for everyone, and besides, the output you get from a pump is not necessarily reflective of how much milk your baby drains from a breast. The other thing I had going for me in addition to a bountiful supply was that I'd never experienced mastitis. I certainly spent enough time worrying about it, but I never actually had it.

I pumped exclusively for six months, and my husband was completely supportive of whatever I wanted to do. At night, we worked out a routine where Stella would wake, he would prepare and feed her a bottle, and I would pump for the next feed. I had two sets of bottles and tubing, so I could wash one lot (or put everything in a big plastic bag in the fridge) and then the next lot of paraphernalia was ready to go.

After six or seven months I'd had enough. I was skinnier than I was before I'd had the baby and deeply exhausted. Once Stella was on the move it became too difficult to pump and entertain her at the same time. We were also wanting to get pregnant again, and I had a hunch (which turned out to be true) that I'm one of those women whose fertility doesn't return until I stop breastfeeding.

I chose a date and started using the stash of breastmilk from the freezer before moving onto formula for a few months.

MY SECOND BREASTFEEDING EXPERIENCE

Should you try again if you're planning another baby? I don't know. I'm sharing my second story not because I think this is what is right for everyone, it's simply how things were for me. There are a lot of physical and emotional factors that go into deciding whether to breastfeed, chest feed, use formula or donor milk or even something else. You don't need to justify or explain your choices to anyone, and definitely not me! I'm sharing my experience in case it's useful.

My experience with Lily was completely different. By the time I was pregnant again, I was more deeply immersed in birth work. I had more connections; I'd spent more time researching ad reflecting and I was determined to try again. My doula gave me full support and confidence that I'd be able to breastfeed, despite my previous challenges. She introduced me to darling Amberley and we unpacked the whole experience. Things with Amberley were just different. Because she was hired privately, instead of through the hospital, she had time. At that time, she was still doing a few midwife shifts here and there but her passion was being able to offer breastfeeding support full-time. Amberley was the first person who told me I could do this, and I actually believed her.

We met first via a phone consultation when I was around 36 weeks pregnant. The night Lily was born, she came to the hospital and we met properly. She arrived with her knitted boob prop and her dummy baby. We put Lily next to the prop baby and marvelled at just how huge Lily seemed next to this average-sized newborn doll. She was warm and gentle and took her time. There is nothing better than being cared for by a Taurean! My husband is also a Taurean, so between the two of them I felt I had the perfect cheer squad. Amberley remained confident, positive and consistent. She never once doubted me or my baby's ability. That one thing changed everything.

What also helped was that Amberley came to visit me in my own house a couple of times. It was a bit of trek, but she did it. She sent me text messages and voice memos, and I was never left in the situation of being the person who had to reach out to ask for help. She seemed to instinctively understand that new parents are exhausted, can't focus or remember anything and often feel they are in over their heads. I was still terrified a lot of the time. I still had damage that needed healing. I still used a pump, but she knew what to do to support us each step of the way and I never felt rushed. I never felt I was doing something wrong. At around six weeks or so, everything seemed to click and I mostly felt I knew what I was doing, even if it was awkward. I even got the hang of feeding in public, which was previously one of my deepest fears.

WHAT I LEARNT FROM MY OWN EXPERIENCE

From my own two unique breastfeeding experiences, I learned:

There are so many breastfeeding myths and so much negative story-telling handed down through families, friends and healthcare workers alike. Midwives are a mixed bag. Some are great at breastfeeding support, some are not and people's personal opinions have a way of coming in, even when they are not invited.

The language we use is important because it leads to fulfilment of self-fulfilling prophecies and 'proof' for an already overwhelmed mother that she isn't enough.

We can be doing more to teach birthing women about the ways in which certain interventions (medications, scalp clips, caesarean section) may impact breastfeeding.

Learning to express and handle your own boobs before you give birth is a skill we could be teaching more.

We can encourage birthing women to make a breastfeeding plan rather than waiting to get help if things get difficult. Forget all the cutesy shit your baby doesn't either need or care about. Pool together and get your pregnant or expecting friend a lactation consultant. Or get them meals, a doula, a cleaner—anything that is going to make their life easier.

Less than 5 per cent of women actually have insufficient milk supply (due to insufficient glandular tissue). There are many other factors contributing to difficulties with breastfeeding.

The benefits of time and patience. That the breast crawl is replicable for months. If the first time doesn't work out, there's still time to encourage babies to use their instincts.

You can see the handout I used about applying the '4 P' analysis to my breastfeeding history on the website www.doctorerin.com.au/podcast.

If you've experienced breastfeeding trauma, know that you're not alone. There are so many factors that go into it. Again, there's more to it than a healthy baby. Breastmilk is amazing and has many benefits, but don't let anything damage your mental health and feelings of self-worth. It's wonderful to overcome challenges, but a mother and a baby are a dyad. It has to be right for both of them.

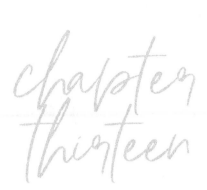

I Don't Even Know if I Like My Baby: Bonding and Attachment

Note: this section uses the word 'mother' frequently. This is because most of the research on infant bonding and attachment has historically looked at the mother-infant dyad. It's important research, but I duly note the language is not as inclusive as it could be.

Is it normal to feel nothing for your baby? To feel like maybe you don't know what all the fuss is about and you're not sure if you even like your baby? Yes!

When Stella was born, I felt happy and calm, but I didn't exactly feel that intense loved-up state that other people talk about. Initially, I put that down to just being a slightly more reserved person. It wasn't until I birthed Lily (unmedicated), and after the fight-or-flight response had dissipated, that I had any idea what people meant by that oxytocin rush.

I didn't exactly feel love while I was in agonising pain after Stella's birth. I didn't exactly feel love when every breastfeeding attempt was painful and I felt like a failure. I distinctly remember the paediatrician coming to visit and engage me in talk about Stella, but I just didn't care. I was in so much pain, I couldn't focus on anything else. In my case, I don't think I felt fully bonded to her until she was no longer the cause of physical pain to my body. It's hard to put on paper, but it is my truth, and if you've felt like this, know that you're not alone.

If you've had a traumatic, painful or scary pregnancy, birth or postpartum experience, this is normal. It's normal for you or your partner to feel anger and resentment at your baby. Particularly on the second night after birth, when babies seem to suddenly realise they are no longer in the womb. They become aware that they are cold, scared, hungry and uncomfortable, so they cry a lot. Adjusting to sleep deprivation is rough. Looking at the clock counting down the minutes to that next painful injury check or breastfeed is normal. Feeling terrified and alienated from your baby who has gone straight to the neonatal intensive care unit is expected.

Remember again that we are emotionally complex. We can be in two or more competing emotional states at once. You can love your baby and still feel a cascade of negative emotions, or even neutral ones.

We are socialised to put all our attention onto the baby after giving birth. Going through one of the most difficult experiences of your life and having people bypass you because you're supposed to be excited about a new baby is confusing. When a new baby is born, I always make an effort to say 'I hope birth went the way you wanted, and if it didn't, I'm thinking of you'. This is because I know what it feels like to have your traumatic experience completely railroaded by another person. As a society, we have far more empathy for the bride whose wedding flowers aren't up to snuff than we do for the woman who has just had a terrifying birth.

We don't talk about birth injuries, blistered boobs and what it felt like to think you were dying because look! There's a baby! Aren't they cute? How much do they weigh, do they look like their dad? Who are they named after? No-one gives a fuck about you and what you've just been through. Or at least that's how it feels.

After Stella was born, we waited a few days to make a public announcement because I wasn't quite ready for the onslaught of positivity. I wanted a few days to attempt to process what the hell had happened to me. I wasn't ready for superfluous things like how much she weighed and who she looked like to overtake the fact that I was lying in bed completely in shock as I received my second blood transfusion. I wanted to be happy, of course, but it felt forced. I refused flat out to have any visitors. As someone who is an introvert living in the countryside, I found the adjustment of having up to 30 different staff members coming in and out of the hospital room in a 24-hour period enough to deal with.

In the past I had sent people the token message 'hope mum and bub are doing well', but very few people actually asked how I was. And to be fair, even if they had asked and were genuinely interested in an honest answer, I probably would have put on a brave face. With my first baby I was so determined to be independent and show people that I was perfectly capable. I now know that people who work in healthcare, especially around childbirth, often have low self-compassion, impostor fears and the feeling that people will judge them. Because we are 'supposed to' know how to do this, right? The person who is doing the worst of the judging is probably you.

Bonding with a baby is not always as instant as we might think, and that's OK. You might need help. Just as birth and breastfeeding are not miraculous things that just happen, the same can be true for bonding. It's often a push–pull relationship in the beginning. With my recovery from surgery and breastfeeding difficulties, there were times when I would welcome my husband taking Stella out of the house so I didn't have to split my attention. But then he'd leave, and I'd feel a wave of guilt, shame and panic, and beg him to turn around and come back.

Taking some time to get to know this new stranger in your life and having moments of uncertainty are normal. However, if the weeks are turning into months and you're feeling that you're not really bonding with your baby, or don't know how to do it, please reach out and get help. Bonding is sometimes instinctive, and sometimes it's not. Bonding is, however, a teachable skill, and there are people who specialise in parent and infant mental health.

HOW TO BOND WITH YOUR BABY

Just as in any relationship, you'll have periods of time where you are connected and your faces and bodies are close, but you'll also need time for breaks from each other. Effective bonding doesn't mean that you need to be in each other's faces all the time! In fact, new babies can become overstimulated easily, as lots of neural activity in their brains is taking place, and it is tiring. With practise, you can learn the cues that your baby does or does not want to connect with you right now.

When babies want to connect, they:
- Smile, search for your face, and look into your eyes.
- May make little noises like coos or laughs, and will look bright and interested.

Activities to connect with your baby might include:
- Touch and cuddles. Skin-to-skin if you can. Take your baby to bed and just spend some time with your baby against you. Or stroke your baby's face and hands.
- Responding when your baby cries. Taking a deep breath when it feels uncomfortable and you don't know why your baby is crying. Creating a trusting relationship where your child can cry and feel safe with you is the long-term goal. You don't have to know why your baby is crying all the time.
- Talking to your baby in soothing, reassuring tones. This helps your baby learn to recognise the sound of your voice. It will also help them learn language. You can talk about anything. Explain what you're doing and what you see.
- Singing songs. Babies typically like up-and-down tunes as well as rhythm. Singing can also help you to slow down and take some regulated breaths.
- Looking into your baby's eyes while you talk and sing, and making facial expressions. This is the one person you can truly be yourself around without being embarrassed or self-conscious, so embrace it.

When your baby needs a break, they might:
- Turn their head away, close their eyes or yawn. They might squirm, pull away, clench their fists or tense their body and cry.
- When this happens, you can place your baby down next to you, and sit together without the intense eye contact. You can place them in a safe place, or pop them in a baby carrier and go to the toilet or make a cup of tea. It's ok to take a break from each other. This is how we integrate new memories and learning.

When you need a break, but your baby is crying:
- Place your baby somewhere safe and take a moment to take some breaths. Leaving a baby to cry for a minute is better than transferring your rage and intense emotions to your baby.
- If you are really worked up, move away from your baby, go into another room and scream into a pillow. Let all the rage and tension leave your body.
- Call one of the people on your safety plan.
- If there is no-one nearby to help, try putting your baby in a carrier and walking around or popping them in the pram. Use movement to release some of that pent-up energy in a way that's safe and healthy.
- Absolutely every parent has days like these. If they are happening regularly, and you're just not feeling any joy, or getting any sleep, ask for help. There is no gold medal that gets handed out for being the parent who never needed any help. We simply cannot function in isolation.

WHY PEOPLE STRUGGLE WITH BONDING

Making sure that your baby has an emotionally and physically supportive caregiver is incredibly important for their health and development. So why might you be struggling?

There are a few reasons. With a significant mental health problem like trauma, depression or psychosis, your emotions, facial expressions and ability to interact with your baby might be flattened, heightened or disorganised. You might be grieving the loss of other babies or family members, or you may have chronic pain. It might also be that your own early childhood experiences and relationships with your parents or care providers are impacting on your ability to feel safe and secure in this new relationship with a baby. I've said before that having a child is like holding a mirror up to yourself where you are forced to look at things about yourself that you'd rather not deal with. It is amazing just how much having our own children can trigger our own childhood experiences.

SECURE AND INSECURE ATTACHMENT TYPES

If you've never learned about different attachment styles and how they might impact your relationships (including with your baby), this might be helpful information. Wherever there is a difficulty in any relationship within your family or with intimate relationships or friendships, going back to attachment styles as a frame of reference can be helpful. Note that loving someone and having a secure attachment are not the same thing. You can love someone, but still not completely trust them or feel safe with them. Let's explore the different types of attachments.

SECURE ATTACHMENT

In an ideal world, all of us would feel secure in our relationships. In general, most people have a healthy, secure attachment style. This means they are comfortable with intimacy, can trust someone when they are out of sight, and generally feel satisfied. They can relax in relationships.

A secure, healthy relationship with one or both parents is important. It means that we can go and explore the world as children, but also feel safe and protected. In secure infant–parent attachments, a baby will look to their parent for comfort when they are hungry, scared or uncertain. A securely attached infant will be wary of strangers and new things, but look to their parent or caregiver to see how they react. When they are old enough to see themselves as separate from their primary caregiver, they will fuss if that parent leaves the room. However, they will generally settle in the knowledge that their caregiver can be trusted and will come back (outside of peak separation anxiety periods, which are normal).

In adulthood, someone who has experienced secure attachments loves their partner, but still has their own identity. They know what it is to let someone out of their sight and know that they are still safe and so is the other person. Secure people have often seen direct examples of peaceful conflict resolution in relationships. They generally don't sabotage their relationships. They accept and have empathy for their partner's shortcomings, and are responsive to the partner's needs. Even in conflict, they are generally well equipped to make their points while listening to their partner without getting personal. Note here, of course, that it is possible to have experienced secure attachments in childhood and yet end up with relationships that do not have this same honesty and trust.

INSECURE ATTACHMENT

There are other attachment styles that are less optimal, and can lead to difficulties with social and emotional development. There are different terms used to describe them, but I'll focus on anxious/ambivalent, anxious/avoidant and anxious/disorganised attachment types. Insecure attachments are a typical response to childhood trauma. Now, what's important to note before you read on is that having the experience of a traumatic birth does not automatically mean you'll have difficulties with attachment. Insecure attachments are more likely to form in response to an accumulation of chronic trauma.

Anxious attachments happen when parents may be unpredictable and inconsistent in their caregiving and empathy. When I've met clients with an anxious/ambivalent attachment style, they often have difficulty expressing their emotions in a healthy way. They might feel clingy towards people, stand-offish or unsure if they can ever trust anyone. They might do things like hide their true feelings, or feel like they need to escalate their emotions and reactions in order to get other people's love and attention. They have typically had one or more parents who were unpredictable. Maybe sometimes Mum met their needs and responded with love and empathy, but other times she was aloof, cold, explosive or somehow made the experience about her. They may also have experienced a parent who was absent, disappearing and reappearing and being inconsistent with their involvement in the child's life.

Anxious/avoidant attachments sometimes happen when a parent is intolerant of emotions, or thinks that successful parenting is about being authoritarian and punitive. These children might be punished for simply being children—making too much noise, or showing too much emotion. The children then feel fearful of the parent and quickly learn to avoid showing feelings in order to stay safe. As adults, they may avoid intimacy, conceal their emotions, and disengage whenever there is conflict. They might have black and white views about 'good' versus 'bad' emotions, or unchallenged beliefs about negative emotions being useless, excessive or unhealthy.

Anxious/disorganised attachments are not discussed as much in everyday discussions about attachment theory, because they are rare. This attachment style usually represents severe trauma and/ or neglect. For example, let's say there is a baby who is placed in an orphanage where there is overcrowding, poor staff training and low resources. This baby may be placed in a cot alone for a large part of the day and night. Staff may be abusive, absent or simply thinking they are doing the right thing by being aloof and not getting too attached. The baby then becomes fearful and anxious about the person whom they rely on to keep them alive. This creates a conflict which completely disorganises the baby's identity, emotions and ability to cope. The continued experience of fear without the resolution of love and safety has the brain compensate by trying to avoid all social interactions. These babies often show behaviours such as shutting down and showing no emotions at all, and they rely on themselves or objects to provide stimulation and soothing. Some will bang their heads, bite their hands and develop other obsessive 'stimming' behaviours in an attempt to soothe their nervous system.

These attachment styles are formed early in life, before we can even communicate our stress with words. Continually feeling anxious without resolution leads to high levels of stress. Our adrenal glands kick in and adrenaline and cortisol are produced. The resting heart rate increases, blood pressure goes up, and we stay in an 'alert and alarmed' state rather than a 'rest and digest' state. When this state happens frequently, it is sometimes referred to as toxic stress. This constant state of stress impacts the development of a child's brain and weakens the immune system. Toxic stress has the ability to switch on the expression of genes which can impact our health much later in life. There's also growing evidence that it can impact the health of future generations of our families.

How Do We Measure Attachment?

The 'strange situation' experiment is an oldie, but a goodie. A mother and one-year old child will typically play together in a room while experimenters watch behind one-way glass and observe and record what they see. After a few minutes, the mother will leave the room and the child will be left alone. The key to measuring attachment is not in how the child reacts when she leaves, but how they react when she returns. Securely attached children will typically greet their mother with a smile, a hug and will seem happy that she has returned. They will settle and eventually get back to playing. Children with an insecure attachment style can be ambivalent or avoidant about their mother returning. It's as if they are bracing themselves to see what emotions and behaviours she will demonstrate because history has taught them that they can't consistently rely on a warm, safe response. Some will be inconsolable, unable to stop crying, and will not re-engage with play. Others might appear completely uninterested in whether their mother is present or not.

THE 'STILL FACE' EXPERIMENT

There are decades of research that have been dedicated to this experiment. In brief, a mother and her baby, usually around 12 months old, is brought into a research lab. The mother is asked to play and interact with her baby in the way that they usually do, while experimenters observe and code the interactions they see. The mother and baby greet each other, smile and coordinate their emotions and intentions about what they want. Then the experimenters will ask the mother to suddenly not respond to the baby, but keep her face still. The baby quickly picks up on this and then will do whatever they can to get their mother to re-engage with them. They smile, point, verbalise, screech, cry, then turn away and become distressed and confused. After this period of a blank face lasting for about two minutes, the mother re-engages with and soothes her baby. It doesn't sound very pleasant, but it's an experiment that's been repeated many, many times with the same results. It shows how in tune babies are with their primary caregivers, and how important a strong emotional and physical bond is in the early years of life.

BABIES CAN TELL IF YOU ARE LYING OR TRYING TO CONCEAL EMOTIONS

Research from Concordia University in Montreal has shown that if you hurt yourself and try to laugh your way through the pain, a baby aged 18 months can tell that you're lying.[27] Or, to put it another way, they are able to pick up on 'unjustified' or mismatched emotional responses such as laughing despite experiencing pain. Try it yourself. You'll need a high chair, a toy ball, and the assistance of an adult who knows your baby well. Place your baby (aged 15 to 20 months) in the high chair and pantomime the following two scenes:

> Using a hammer or an object that mimics a hammer, pretend to tinker around before acting as if you had accidentally hit your finger with the hammer. Ouch! Wince and make appropriate faces, holding your expression until your baby looks away.

> The other adult will hand you a ball. Express boredom until you get the ball. Then, look at the ball with excitement and give a big smile. Again, hold your expression until your baby looks away.

A few days later, repeat the two scenes, but this time, switch around the emotional responses, so smile after hitting yourself with the hammer and grimace when you're handed the ball.

At age 15 months, the hypothesis is that your baby is not likely to respond differently to the justified and unjustified emotional responses. They will probably respond to sad face (justified or unjustified) by showing a sad or concerned facial expression in return. However, from around 18 months old, if you show an infant an unjustified response (smiling after hitting yourself with a hammer) your baby probably won't be fooled. They will probably spend more time looking at you to check out what's going on and respond with empathy to your pain even if you're smiling.

Adults tend to want to shield infants from distress by putting on a brave or happy face following a negative experience, but this research seems to suggest that this technique really only works with younger babies.

It also seems that babies around this age are quick to work out whether an adult is reliable or not. In a scenario similar to the one above, the researchers played a game with an empty box. They firstly primed the babies to think that an adult was reliable or unreliable. To create an 'unreliable' adult, the experimenter would look inside a container while expressing excitement. When the baby looked in the box, they would see that it was empty. In contrast, for the 'reliable' adult group, the baby would look into the box and see a toy.

Later, they had the babies watch the same adult use their forehead instead of their hand to turn on a light. The experimenters then waited to see which babies would copy the behaviour. More than half of the babies who had watched the 'reliable' adult copied them by trying to turn the light on with their forehead. For the other group, it seems that the babies knew that the adult had lied to them before, so were a lot less likely to copy their behaviour.

Attachment theory psychologist John Bowlby is often quoted as saying 'What cannot be communicated to the mother cannot be communicated to the self', meaning that people with insecure attachments have difficulty understanding themselves and communicating their needs and wants to other people.

The goal of this chapter on bonding and attachment is not to have you panic, but to help you do some reflection about your relationship with your baby and with other people. It's to reassure you that bonding is a learning process and that it's OK if you recognise that you need help.

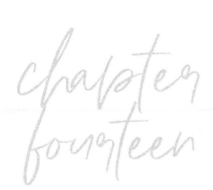

'It Didn't Happen to You, So Shut Up': Vicarious Trauma in Partners

Birth trauma impacts at least one in three birthing women, but who is often left out of the picture? The partners. Vicarious trauma in birthing partners is very real, and yet there is little to no acknowledgement, let alone resources to help.

Witnessing birth trauma as a partner has the potential to: (1) create severe cognitive dissonance ('I know what happened to my partner was wrong, yet I did nothing to stop it'), (2) contribute to unresolved feelings of shame, guilt, helplessness and rage, and/or difficulties with bonding, (3) contribute to heightened nervous system activity (e.g. oscillating between 'fight' mode and 'freeze' mode), and (4) contribute to an unhelpful, negative birth storytelling culture which minimises the role of partners.

On the other hand, partners who are well supported emotionally, cognitively and socially have phenomenal potential for growth. In this chapter, I want to provide validation and education for the very real effects of vicarious trauma. I also want to explore what it means to work with partners through the lens of post-traumatic growth and how to validate and educate about trauma in a way that allows partners to step into self-compassion. We will explore how to inspire partners to see their own potential for growth, leadership and even advocacy.

THE ROLE OF PRE-EXISTING TRAUMA

When you walk into a birth space, you are bringing all your past traumas with you. This is something that is more frequently discussed with the birthing woman. Care providers might ask about possible abuse or previous traumas that could impact a birthing woman's ability to feel safe. However, partners are not typically prompted to consider how their own traumas might impact how they feel in the birth space—unless of course you are someone who is fully aware that you already experience multiple microaggressions daily (e.g. partners who identify as LGBTQI, Indigenous and/or in an ethnic minority).

Pre-existing traumas can include assault, abuse, bullying, accidents, injuries or previous negative experiences of being in hospital, among other events. They can also mean realising that you don't look like the shiny people on the hospital brochure. It can mean the experience of not being sure if you are welcome in a hospital or other setting. It can mean being called by the wrong pronoun, or having someone make assumptions about your identity or role in the birth. Already feeling uneasy, unwelcome, invisible or unsafe in the birth space can open the possibility for further trauma.

NEGATIVE BIRTH BIAS

British singer Robbie Williams once famously said that watching his wife give birth was 'like watching your favourite pub burning down'. We also frequently hear stories of men coaching other men who are preparing for birth by advising them to 'stay at the top end'. My husband James was one of them. I used to tell all my hypnobirthing couples that before I trained in hypnobirthing, James used to joke about waiting until we could have a baby in a can, meaning that we should wait until such as time as science and technology had progressed far enough that we could grow our baby in artificial womb. He consumed an awful lot of science fiction as a teenager! I share this story because we were those overeducated science-loving people who thought that as technology progressed, this would automatically make birth safer. We were socialised to believe that birth was dangerous, scary and gross.

Most partners who are raised as men in the West are not given a great deal of positive imagery or storytelling about birth. If you were born in the 1980s or even the 90s in Australia, it's likely that your own dad didn't attend your birth. He may have been pacing around the hallway smoking a Winnie Blue and waiting for the cricket scores. OK, that is a gross generalisation but hopefully you see the point I'm trying to make. What we are told about birth, the images, the emotions and the storytelling (or absence of it) impacts how we show up in birth.

VICARIOUS TRAUMA

'Oh, but I'm not the one who went through it, so it's not as bad.'

If you are a partner, family member or care provider like a midwife or doula, saying this to yourself, let's call bullshit on this right now.

I'll give you the same example I've been giving to clients for years. Let's say you are a parent. Wouldn't you rather take a bullet for your child than watch them being shot? I have met adults who have thrown themselves on children using their bodies as a shield during tragic shootings. I have met someone who had to leave children inside their burning house because it was too late and too unsafe to go in. The conflict of wanting to rescue them, yet knowing you have a partner who still needs you, is a no-win situation.

I've said it before, and I'll say it again. Humans are complex. We can be in two (or more) equal or competing emotional states at once. It doesn't mean that we need to start classifying, comparing or ranking them—except that this is exactly what we do when we are under threat.

When there is a current threat, ranking and comparing information is an important skill. If you're walking along and suddenly a gigantic bear sneaks out from behind a rock then your brain might go straight into classifying and ranking 'How far away is the bear?' and 'Where can I run to?' and 'What kind of bear is it? A baby? Or an angry mother bear?'. When the threat has passed, however, the comparing and ranking are no longer serving us. It becomes more helpful to think of the family as a unit. What does everyone need? Partners included.

WHAT IS THE BYSTANDER EFFECT?

When I'm working with partners or teaching birth workers, I always like to start by normalising the experience of the bystander effect in birth trauma for what it is—fucked up! If you've never heard of the bystander effect before, it's a phenomenon where people who are watching a tragedy unfold sometimes fail to step in and help but instead stand around and watch. Part of the theory suggests that the more people there are, the more likely that empathy turns into apathy. You've likely seen it before—either in real life or on the news. Someone passes out in the street and people stand around and watch.

It happens in birth all the time. A room can suddenly fill with people, and you feel invisible, in the way or useless. Even if you want to help, social rules and the pecking order of hospital staff dictate that you don't. For partners, this can be extremely traumatic and confusing. It creates a conflict that the brain cannot find resolution with.

In what other setting would you watch your partner in pain, maybe held down, cut open, handled roughly and spoken to rudely, and you stand back and don't even say anything? Your instinct says to fight or flee, but your rational brain says you must stay back and let the experts take over. Or you simply freeze up.

It challenges people at the very core of what they value and who they believe themselves to be, yet the power of social rules and conditioning teaches us to suppress those primal instincts to protect. Look at the Milgram experiment—people willingly being convinced to electrocute someone because a researcher told them to. Or the Stanford Prison Experiment—people torturing and humiliating people for science because they are conditioned to believe that they are superior. We can condition people to behave in ways that they wouldn't normally.

GENDER DIFFERENCES IN COPING

Now I want to add a caution to this discussion about male and female differences in coping. Most of the research on couples is on heterosexual couples. Please take it very generally. We still have a long way to go before the research is more representative of LGBTQI folks, including trans, questioning and intersex. Looking at gender differences in coping is just one way of exploring the birth trauma experience for partners. I fully acknowledge that the following passage might not sit right with your experiences and doesn't represent your voice.

Remember in Chapter 4 where I talked about the different styles of coping? I don't want to go too 'Men are from Mars, women are from Venus' here, but there are merits to looking at the ways in which gender influences coping. The gist of coping research as it applies to gender is that women typically seek out emotion-focused coping. They use social support, venting, talking and sharing emotions without the expectation that the other person 'fixes it'.

Men instead often listen through the emotions for the pragmatic 'problem' and want to find a practical solution. This is known as solution-focused coping—Googling answers to questions, research, reading, trying to come up with a five-point plan and a pro-and-con list.

This is super, super general, but over time I've found that this explanation in coping differences can help couples figure out why they are not in sync when it comes to facing challenges. If you've heard of the five love languages by Gary Chapman (useful to know about yourself, your partner and your kids), you could see coping in a similar way. There's a basic menu of options, but we each have our favourites and we can become so ingrained in our own version of reality that we forget that not everyone shares our preferences.

Something I have seen fairly often in birth professional groups is where someone asks 'What support is there for birth partners after trauma?'. People (usually women!) will then go into a long laundry list of things that *they* would want. It is easy to forget that just because you, your client and other people you know share similar coping styles this doesn't mean that this is what someone else wants or needs. Not everyone wants to talk about their trauma and use emotion-focused coping. This is partially why eye movement desensitisation and reprocessing (EMDR), which doesn't involve as much talking about the trauma as say CBT, is frequently used as first-line treatment for male veterans.

WORKING WITH RELUCTANT PARTNERS

Another common questions I get is 'How do I make my partner get help?'. The answer to this is simple: you can't! We must consider the old chestnut about leading a horse to water; you simply can't make someone get help, even if you think they need it. That's not how behaviour change works.

I have spent part of my career attempting to work with people who have been forced to get help. People in the criminal justice system who've been mandated to receive anger, parenting or drug and alcohol support. People who have been mandated to seek counselling or other skills from their workplace or registration board. Children, teenagers and adults who simply don't want to be there. While it's not impossible to win people over and convince them to do things they don't want to do (I've had some success!), people who are 'made' to seek support do not engage. This can activate feelings of failure and anger and seeing therapy as a waste of time. For both of us, actually.

The only real exception to this in mental health is when someone is 'sectioned' or subject to the Mental Health Act. This means that someone's behaviour or current mental state is so dangerous to themselves or someone else that they lose control over their own decisions. An example might be someone who has anorexia and is literally going to die if someone doesn't step in and force them to take in nourishment. Even then, people sometimes tragically find ways to pull feeding tubes out, block them or end their life in some other way.

UNDERSTANDING WHY PARTNERS WON'T GET HELP

There needs to be some motivation (internal or external) for seeking support that is meaningful to the individual. What you're suggesting must be:

- valued
- aligned with their world view
- measurable and achievable
- and, ideally, consistent with and valued by their social group.

The stages of change model refers to a specific series of stages that

people pass and repass through when deciding to change their
behaviour:

- pre-contemplation (I call this the 'not interested in
  what you're selling' stage). In this stage there is zero
  recognition of a problem, and no intent to change in the
  next six to 12 months.
- contemplation (I call this 'window shopping'). They may
  or may not be convinced to think about change in the
  next six months. They are at least sitting on the fence.
- preparation ('credit card at the ready'). They are
  interested in change and in the process of committing
  to action.
- action ('made a purchase'). They are actively and
  successfully taking steps to change their behaviour.
- maintenance ('enjoying the purchase'). They are
  keeping up the good work, feeling more confident, and
  continuing to see the results of positive change.
- relapse ('I lost or broke the purchase'). A setback. They
  have temporarily regressed to old behaviours and
  patterns. We then reassess their motivation to change
  again, and go back through the loop.

Behaviour change is effective when people are at least cycling
between the contemplation, preparation and action stages. Many
people (experienced therapists included) make the mistake of
assuming that attending an appointment means someone is in the
contemplation stage. Not at all. Almost all therapy interactions
involve working your way through the stages of change model
(and back and forth) several times. If someone is not interested
(pre-contemplation), there are definitely things that we can do to
try to convince them, but we must remember their circumstances
and maintain our respect for individual differences.

When someone is pre-contemplative about seeking support, and you really think they need it, you might just start by sharing what you observe without judging: 'I see you staying up late', 'I hear you changing the subject when I try to talk about the birth'.

You can make resources available—books, websites and so on. You can appeal to commonsense analogies: if you broke your leg would you put up with it? If your child was sick or having trouble wouldn't you want support? If you knew you needed to learn a skill wouldn't you go and get skills training? You can remind them that coping is a learnt skill. If your parents or school or friends had never taught you how to drive, would you just put up with it or would you find someone who could teach you? Would you blame yourself for not being able to fully teach yourself or would you accept that for some things you need assistance?

You can share the fact that support can mean more than talking about emotions. Many people are unaware that there are options other than talking and reflecting. Again, EMDR and other approaches for trauma don't focus on talking at all.

16 TRIES TO DECIDE

It feels weird to end with a marketing analogy, but as I get older, the more I see that before you can be an effective teacher, healer or advocate, you need to be a bloody good marketer. If you have children, learning to convince people to listen to you and let you guide them is a sales exchange. I read somewhere that it takes 12 touch points to make a sale. I have no idea who said it, or if the number is accurate. The point is that people are unlikely to buy what you're trying to sell upon the first try.

If the marketing analogy isn't working for you, let's use something more tangible. I once watched a documentary on fussy eating, and the psychologist featured (Catherine Dendy) explained that it takes 16 tries to decide if you even like a food. Being a scientist, I tried it out on myself. Previously, I've been someone who hates coriander, asparagus and rocket. With persistence and repeated exposure I can now eat those things and actually enjoy them. Note that this might not work for everyone! Food preferences and the ability to tolerate tastes and textures are way more complicated than that. I still cannot tolerate aniseed or liquorice. The point is that maybe with repeated exposure and gentle, respectful encouragement you might convince your partner to seek support. However, you might not and that has to be OK. Not everyone likes liquorice and you can't make them!

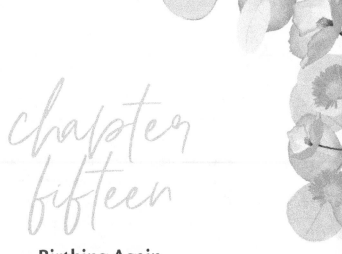

Birthing Again
(When You're Shit Scared)

'I don't think I can do this again.'

Ah yes, the phrase I uttered in those first few hours after my first birth. As if that's the time to be making decisions, prioritising and even thinking about another baby!

I know that for some people, the experience of birth has the opposite effect. They say they can't wait to give birth again. I was 35 when a midwife friend told me the 'real reason' people knock before entering your room in hospital. And the real reason there's a curtain around your hospital bed. Maybe, like me you've assumed it's for your privacy and modesty getting in and out of bed, feeding and so on. Yeah, it's because some people have sex straight after birth. The adrenaline, oxytocin vibes, and in some cases, cultural or other expectations, have people starting the cycle again. Everyone is different.

After my miscarriage, my husband and I knew we wanted to try again straight away. I don't mean straight after the D&C, but within a few weeks we were both ready. That shocked some people. I'm not sure where the whole 'you have to wait three months' rule came from, but my healthcare provider told me it was fine. In fact, I'd read that your body can actually be at its most fertile after a miscarriage, and I know several people who have conceived very quickly after one. Six weeks after my D&C, I was pregnant with Stella. About six months after she was born, we were ready for another baby.

If you're contemplating another pregnancy, or actively trying to cope with one, this is the section where I'll suggest some things to think about differently with birth—remembering that every birth, baby and parent is different. Remembering that you can do all the research and planning, have a positive mindset and an amazing birth team, and still have a traumatic birth. That again, there is no 'just be more positive next time' or 'hire a doula and everything will be fine'.

Let me also just say that if your traumatic birth ended in infant loss, I honour you. If you have decided not to have more babies, or had that decision taken away from you, I honour you. I want to acknowledge how quick we are to ask people when they are having the next baby. That they ask this question completely discounting severe birth injuries, disability, secondary infertility, trauma, postpartum mental illness and the psychological toll of sleep deprivation.

So, I've spent hundreds of hours thinking about this—thinking about how could I identify exactly what I did during and after my traumatic births to end up coping OK. Did I have a lot of training in mental health and coping? Yes. Am I just a resilient person? Maybe. But I honestly believe coping is a learned skill. A teachable skill. And when you have the skills to teach others to improve humanity, then you must share them. So, here are a few things I did that I can order into a set of teachable skills.

FINE ACRONYM

This is what I teach about how people can protect themselves from developing trauma reactions. It's not a prescription. It's not about saying 'if you do these things, you'll be fine', but it helped me (and an acronym helps you remember!).

F: BEING FUTURE-FOCUSED

People who can find some hope and remain future-focused during a traumatic event do tend to cope better than people who get stuck on ideas of hopelessness. The technical term for this is activating your dorsolateral cortex. When I was birthing Lily, I kept repeating to myself 'I'm OK', 'I'm going to get through this', 'it will only be another minute'. I also had silent conversations with my baby 'come on, baby, we're OK', and 'we can do this'.

In contrast, those people who panic, lose all hope and get stuck in the 'I'm trapped', 'I can't get out', 'I'm doomed' mode of thinking tend to stay stuck. Even though they logically know the trauma has passed, their brain and nervous system keep them stuck in a never-ending loop of panic.

I: INTEGRATE THE INFORMATION

Your brain wants to put things into a story. It's how we process information. It wants a beginning, a middle and an end. It wants a hero who conquers a problem and preferably a parable or a meaning we can extract from it. Marketers and people in advertising use this tactic all the time because they know that the human brain naturally seeks out and pays attention to stories. Remember, the brain directs us to lean into simplicity and lean out from confusion.

Telling a story is not the same as finding out all the information, it's just about creating some kind of narrative that makes sense so your brain can stop firing off random pieces of unconnected information. You might also think of it like editing. Part of any good story telling is editing. Many of the world's most-loved novels and films have gone through several rounds of edits to tighten up the plot, progress characters and clean up miscellaneous and unnecessary details. Nothing is set in stone. Your brain will get used to a new story or new characters. Your draft version of a broken woman can be re-edited into a strong warrior. It's your story. You choose the hero, the journey and the meaning.

N: New Baby Smell

No matter what kind of birth you have, the MRI research shows that smelling your baby activates oxytocin and prolactin, which help turn down the cortisol and adrenaline.[28] [29] Even if you've had loads of drugs or a caesarean section, you don't feel a thing and there's no obvious buzz, do it anyway because the research shows it's still lighting up the pleasure centre of your brain. I also recommend taking lots of photos and videos of that interaction so you can access the muscle memory for it later. After Lily's birth I took a few videos of me sniffing, hugging and kissing her, because that's what I wanted my brain to focus on rather than the trauma. Later, if you're away from your baby and need to pump breastmilk, watching these videos, or looking at photos of your baby and smelling their clothes, can help your milk to let down. It also helps when you miss your child or you're having a rough time with your kids. It can take your brain back to a time of happy, loved-up bliss. As I said, even if you can't feel a thing, do it anyway.

E: ENGAGE SUPPORT

Something from the neck up, like talking to someone. And something from the neck down, like some sort of holistic body support that will help process and integrate trauma stored at a cellular level. Maybe that's yoga, Chinese medicine or embodiment work like somatic experiencing.

Reread the chapter on hormones being your helpers. Build up your oxytocin bank. No matter what kind of birth you plan or what kind of birth you end up having, know that if you've got some spare oxytocin in the bank, it's going to help. Read lots. Take an independent childbirth education course, read books and listen to podcasts about your birth rights.

WHAT'S THE 'RIGHT' CHOICE FOR A SUBSEQUENT BIRTH?

There isn't one! Being able to calmly meet whatever turn your birthing takes (a phrase from Hypnobirthing Australia) will set you up well. For me, that means reading what I need to know to feel informed and empowered. Know your birth rights and get a sense of what is preference versus policy versus the law. It means not going down a rabbit hole and reading too much, though. I think if I'd done loads of research about inductions before my first birth then I might have been more scared, and not coped as well. Similarly the research about 'big' babies or babies born after 42 weeks. For me, there was a sweet spot between feeling informed and feeling overwhelmed. There's going to be a different sweet spot for everyone.

For both my births I wanted as little intervention as possible. Which meant a physiological birth, free from drugs. That might not be what you want or what you need.

If you are survivor of abuse, if you have birth injuries, or other reasons (that you actually don't have to explain to anyone!), a caesarean section might be perfect. I encourage you to read and listen to stories of people who have experienced a wide range. A great place to start is with January Harshe. She is a mum to six kids. She's had caesarean sections, vaginal birth after a caesarean, hospital births, home births, traumatic births and non-traumatic births. Her book *Birth without Fear* is a wealth of information and support for anyone who is giving birth and their support people.

PREPARATION FOR BIRTH: SET AND SETTING

Whether you think you can or you can't—both are right
—Henry Ford

Drug researchers talk about 'set' and 'setting'. Psychedelic or hallucinogenic drugs like LSD, MDMA (ecstasy) and DMT (N-Dimethyltryptamine) are sometimes used in clinical settings to treat depression, anxiety and PTSD. In order for a client to have a safe and useful experience, researchers and practitioners would work carefully to ensure the set and the setting were right for the client.

'Set' is the mental state someone brings to an experience: their thoughts, beliefs (challenged and unchallenged), mood and expectations.

When I taught hypnobirthing, and I was regularly asked 'does it work?', my answer was always this: yes and no. If you go into hypnosis believing it will work, then it will work. If you go into it thinking it's a load of mumbo jumbo then it won't work.

'Setting' is the physical and social environment. Being with a safe, supportive social group is a huge part of that.

Can you see the similarities with birth? I've said it before, but during birth you really are the most open you'll ever be, physically, emotionally, and spiritually. If the set and setting are calm and supportive, magic can happen. If, on the other hand, the sacred balance of the birth space is thrown off, then the birthing woman (and support people and care providers) may not have a good experience.

MINDSET

Mindset is everything. I'm a big fan of the phrase 'how you do anything is how you do everything'. You've got to believe that you can do this, no matter what turn your birth takes. Your care team and your partner also have to believe in you.

SURRENDER

How are you with this word? How does it feel in your body right now? Surrender is not the same as losing control. Being able to surrender to your body and your baby, to trust them both and take yourself out of your thinking rational brain and slip into your primitive brain, is vital.

Whatever you bring from your childhood, adolescent and early sexual experiences you often bring into birth. If you have a history of experiences where your body has been mistreated, where surrender would have equated to serious injury or death, then just let that sit.

If you've never really been able to orgasm and find it difficult to let go in order to experience sexual pleasure, let that sit. There are many birth researchers who say that birth is a sexual experience.

Again, it's not your fault if you feel unsafe about the word 'surrender'. You're not broken or weak. Birth is a physical experience you can't control. You need to be able to let go and surrender. Being able to fully relax, release and let go—physically, emotionally and spiritually—is the goal. It's also a learnable skill. With support and teaching, you can train for birth just as you would for a marathon.

Keep in mind that the brain doesn't know the difference between what's real and what's imagined. You can retrain anxious, fearful neural pathways with practice. You can do it all just by imagining the positive outcome you want. Think about athletes like gymnasts or racing car drivers. They spend a lot of their time imaging the routine in their mind, training the neural pathways into a deep state of 'knowing'. My father-in-law is a racing car driver and two-time Bathurst winner. Racing cars is very expensive, and it's not practical to get into a V8 or other racing car and practise every day. But what I've seen him do time and time again over the years is watch videos of his races. Memorising the track so his brain overlearns all the turns, dips, corners and places where he can potentially sneak in and push another car out the way!

So again, my recommendation is that you learn hypnosis. Find a hypnobirthing teacher, a hypnotherapist, a psychologist or a birth coach with the appropriate training and skills. Find a doula, independent midwife or other birth attendant who is familiar with hypnosis and can coach you. This is potentially one of the biggest days of your life. Forget all the baby stuff you think you need and invest in yourself.

SAFETY

You need to feel unobserved. Bright lights, loud noises and people in your face are not optimal for releasing birthing hormones. There is a reason that a domestic cat will find a dark, quiet place to birth undisturbed, often in a cupboard.

If homebirth is not an option or not your thing, there is plenty you can do to make a hospital suite feel safer. Hypnobirthing parents often put a sign on the door—'quiet please, we're hypnobirthing'. As simple as it sounds, seeing a sign reminding hospital staff to be quiet before they enter a space can take someone out of autopilot and have them check in with what energy they are bringing into the birthing space.

Turning lights down, closing curtains, moving equipment out of the way (if permitted), covering the clocks and even positioning yourself looking away from the door or medical equipment can help.

Our obsession with numbers in birth (how many minutes was a contraction, how dilated is your cervix, what time is it?) is mostly unhelpful. We have been conditioned to think that these things are more important than they actually are. Michel Odent (and others) explain that the birthing brain doesn't need numbers and language. In fact, asking for and sharing facts and figures takes someone out of their primitive brain and into their rational brain again, which disrupts the flow of hormones.[30] [31]

The World Health Organization now recognise that the unspoken rule that someone in labour should dilate one centimetre every hour is no longer considered useful. Insisting that we do vaginal examinations and check to see dilation is not necessary for most birthing women. You have a right to refuse.

TRUST

You have to be able to trust your care team. You have to be able to trust your baby. You have to be able to trust your body to do this. The last two items in this list are things you can work towards and be taught. The first one can be trickier. If you have the option of choosing your own care provider then be choosy. Interview people, ask about their personal views about birth. Ask about their personal experience with birth. If you don't feel comfortable with them in these meetings, you're unlikely to feel comfortable once you're naked and vulnerable. If you don't have much choice in care provider, then remember you can always ask for a second opinion. You can change provider, even if you're in active labour. You have choices and rights.

I want you to think about all the times you've negotiated a contract. Sent back a coffee or food that wasn't right. Corrected someone if they got your name wrong. Contacted a bank if you were overcharged. Tried to convince your partner that they are wrong about something. You can have difficult conversations. The birth of your baby is not the time to keep quiet and not make a fuss. You are allowed to question people in positions of authority. It's your body and your baby, not theirs. Being able to ask for what you want is one of the most important skills you can learn for yourself. Sit with this, reflect on it, and again, think about where you might have blocks or unchallenged ideas.

YOUR SUBCONSCIOUS

Again, my recommendation is always going to be to take a hypnobirthing class, take an online course or work one-to-one with a coach or psychologist who specialises in hypnobirthing and hypnosis for childbirth. Not all programs are created equal (in my opinion). Some are potentially a bit preachy with 'natural birth or nothing' undertones. Some have male voices on their recordings, some have female. Some focus on numbers and counting while you breathe, some don't. Do your research first to see what might suit you.

You'll find the one that meets your needs best, but if I'm asked, then Hypnobirthing Australia is the program I've personally used and taught, and I know it inside and out. In saying that, I also have friends and clients who have had amazing things to say about other programs. I have dear friends who teach other programs.

Things to consider when choosing a program:

Is it actually independent childbirth education? If it's run in a hospital, your teacher might be restricted in what they can and can't say.

What's the overall view of birth, and what messages are used? I once had a mate tell me she 'failed' hypnobirthing. That's out of alignment with what I teach. As I mentioned, some programs are a bit heavy-handed on the 'natural or nothing' approach. You should not be made to feel that a physiological birth without drugs and intervention is the only 'right' way to birth. In fact, if you're recovering from a severe tear, an obstetric fistula or physical or psychological trauma, being pressured into a natural birth could be dangerous.

BIRTH ENVIRONMENT

I went back to the same obstetrician and the same hospital for my second birth. It was also the same obstetrician and the same hospital who assisted me through my miscarriage. Some people might question why on earth you'd choose to go back to the scene of your trauma. If I know anything about trauma and the reasons why people gravitate back to the same behaviours, people and environments, it's that the brain likes that which is familiar. Mine certainly did. I equated familiarity with safety. Better the devil you know than spend the extra brain power scanning a new environment for threat. I already knew where the exits were, so to speak. I knew I'd looked down the barrel of death (as it was in my view) and come out OK, so I trusted I would be OK again. This is not at all to say that this is what you should do.

I had thought about a home birth, but I had a huge block around the idea of something going wrong and having to wait to receive help. We lived an hour from the hospital (with no traffic) and the idea of having to move or wait for extra assistance if I needed it didn't sit right. My instinct said I would feel safer in a hospital.

Sliding doors, right? Every now and then I'll see someone on Instagram who birthed a big baby at home, no problems, even with shoulder dystocia. There's a wistful 'Oh, maybe I could have done that?', even though I've also heard horror stories. Every time I share my shoulder dystocia birth on social media, I'll get a message from someone saying that I was 'lucky'. That they and/or their baby have injuries. That they lost their baby. There are few circumstances in birth with zero risk.

But who is to say that if I'd hired an experienced midwife, I couldn't have birthed fine at home, even with a huge baby? The more I've researched and read, the more I sometimes wonder if the intervention my baby and I received for shoulder dystocia was necessary. Or was it priming? Is it possible my birth team expected it to happen, so it happened? Or, maybe that's total wishful thinking, and it really was an emergency. I don't know, and I'll never know. The point I want to make here is not to get stuck in analysis paralysis of what might have or will happen.

Clearly if you felt unsafe, if there was negligence and abuse and you didn't like the environment or the care team you had, then change it for next time. Just because I chose to go back to the hospital and doctor that were familiar to me does not mean I think that you should. Sit in meditation, in hypnosis or just in quiet time, and ask yourself 'What do I want?'. Listen for the answer. Try not to force it, just see what happens.

To end this chapter, the most loving advice I could pass on would be to keep repeating the mantra 'different pregnancy, different baby, different day, different outcome'. Because ultimately, that is the truth. It will be different. You can't control the different. If you can't get yourself to really, truly believe that birth will be better, then stick to what is the neutral truth. The next birth will be different, that is for sure.

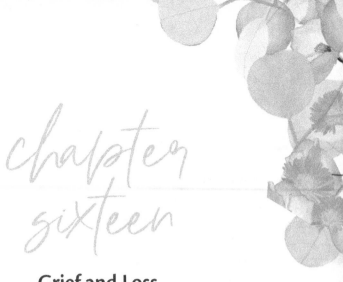

chapter sixteen

Grief and Loss

Nature never hurries, yet everything is accomplished
—LAO TZU

You might be tempted to skip this chapter, telling yourself that this chapter is only for people who lost a baby or their birth partner. While I definitely wanted to dedicate a chapter for people who have experienced death, I'd encourage you to think more broadly. With the journey from maiden to mother to crone (or non-parent to parent) there is loss, death and grief. Honouring what has been lost is a huge part of trauma work. To get you started, let's think about some of the possible experiences of loss and grief you might have:

Loss of self.

Loss of plans (e.g. how you would bring your baby into the world, when you'd bring your baby home, where your baby would sleep).

Loss of your physical body, that is no longer your own (e.g. your hair falls out from hormone changes, your breasts change shape and size, your belly isn't the same anymore, you leak urine and/or faeces after birth).

Loss of control—over choices, outcomes, your body, your emotions.

Loss of income.

Loss of being right, of being able to be logical, do research and find answers to problems.

Grieving the end of your time alone with your partner.

Grieving loss of sleep and adjustment to a chaotic new rhythm.

Loss of friendships.

Grieving the end of birth support relationships (realising that you won't see your obstetrician, midwife or doula anymore).

Loss of support (e.g. when your partnership dissolves, your partner has to go back to work or your family can't be with you).

Grieving the loss of your own parent in a whole new way, now that you are a parent.

There's loads more, of course; this was just a short list to get you thinking.

AN EXERCISE TO PROCESS LOSS

Something you might want to try to process trauma, grief and loss is therapeutic letter writing. I like this exercise because it allows you to brain dump and express yourself fully without being interrupted or filtering.

SET UP

Have time alone, uninterrupted. Preferably with pen and paper. This is the primary way that most of us learned to express ourselves in written form, so it's a less cognitively loaded task. You're less likely to get distracted by spelling and typos, and there are no alerts or other things calling for your attention.

Turn off your phone and all distractions.

Choose *who* and *what* you want to express and release.

Read it aloud for even more power.

Burn it, put it in the shredder, destroy it while setting the intention to release (not the same as forgiving anyone).

Do not hang onto it!

TYPES OF LETTERS

A big 'Fuck you!' angry letter to your obstetrician, midwife, care team, partner, mother-in-law, maybe even your baby.

A disappointment letter to yourself, your mother, society or anyone who had you believe that birth wasn't supposed to be like this.

A jealousy letter to your friend who got the water birth with no tearing. To your sister who made breastfeeding look easy. To the Instagram influencer with a flat belly postpartum.

A love letter to yourself. Didn't get the support, words of comfort and kindness you wanted from someone else? Learn to give them to yourself.

REPARENTING YOURSELF AND SELF-LOVE

A letter to your baby, expressing all your hopes and dreams. All your guilt, shame, anger and sadness.

THE EXPERIENCE OF DEATH

In Western culture, we are so weird about death and dying that we use all sorts of confusing phrases to mean the same thing. I am someone who likes to be up-front and clear in my communication about death. It might be partially because I have family members with autism, and I have spent my life surrounded by people who struggle with idioms. Clear communication is one of my highest values. I have seen so many children struggle to process and understand death because people were trying to protect them with vague statements like 'passed away' or 'gone to a better place'.

I still remember my mother telling me that our cat, Jenny, had gone to a nursing home, like Grandma. I asked her repeatedly when we could visit and why I couldn't I see her. As an animal lover, I found the idea of a convalescent home for cats appealing as a young child. It still does! By the time my grandmother in the nursing home did die, my parents were clearer with me. At six years old, I understood that Grandma's physical body had been cremated and the ashes of her physical body were now in a black rectangular box. I would pick the box up and talk to her through the screw hole that fastened the sealed box together (I thought it was a microphone). At Christmas, I insisted that Grandma be brought out and sat on the table so she could enjoy Christmas lunch with us, as she always had. I like to think I inspired my family to not feel quite so serious and hung up about death. Perhaps that makes me a strange child, but I am not someone who has ever had a problem speaking openly about death.

Death is a personal experience. Just as I say a birth is traumatic if you say it is, I think a baby is a baby if you say it is. Whether you experienced a 'chemical pregnancy', an early miscarriage, a termination, a late-term miscarriage or a stillbirth, I place no rules on who gets to use the term 'baby' and who doesn't. If that's not what you're comfortable with and you'd rather use other terms, that's fine too.

When grief is not given time and space to be heard and validated, our experiences of grief can become protracted and complex. We go back into measurements and comparisons such as 'I wasn't that far along' or 'I shouldn't complain because I still have a living baby', which are understandable, but not helpful.

There is no need to qualify your experience to determine how much you can grieve, or how long you are supposed to grieve for. Just as people cling to numbers in birth ('I'm only six centimetres dilated') they also cling to numbers in death ('It's been six weeks; shouldn't I feel better now?'). Here is the thing. Grief is not a mental illness. Putting a number on the passing of time isn't helpful. There are no rules. Despite the popularisation of the five stages of grief (denial, anger, bargaining, depression and acceptance), it's a guideline not a policy. There is no five-point plan for how to get through grief without feeling pain. It's a process, and feeling pain is part of that.

Most of my discussions about grief and loss with clients and with psychologists I've supervised over the years have been similar. There's the searching for the 'right' thing to say or do. What is the thing that I could do or say to make this process faster or easier? People sometimes get shitty with me when they hear my answer. There's no shortcut, there's no passing, it just is. Radical acceptance of what is in the now is what helps. I'm not even really a fan of the 'time heals all wounds' type of thinking. There is only now and the ongoing practice of self-compassion in the now.

Physical Ways of Honouring a Baby's Death

Hiring a death doula.

Having your baby photographed by a birth photographer who is experienced with death. There are organisations that will provide special clothing for your baby (e.g. Angel gowns).

Planting a tree.

Buying a star and naming it.

Donating your baby's organs.

Donating to a children's charity.

Sponsoring a child.

Getting a tattoo.

Making a keepsake box or journal.

Buying a special piece of jewellery. You can also have keepsake jewellery made with your baby's hair, your breastmilk or embryo ash. At the time of writing, Amy McGlade (aka the breastmilk queen; formerly baby bee hummingbirds) offered these services.

Setting up your own non-profit organisation or charity.

Again, not an exhaustive list, just a few ideas.

This is a short chapter. Short doesn't necessarily mean simple. By the time you cut out all the clichés, things that people say to fill the space and attempts to make death and grief less horrific, what's left is authenticity. Death and grief are hard. There is no need to 'do' anything with it; I think it's more a practice of 'being' with it. If you are finding that the thoughts are just not letting up, you feel isolated and it is impacting your ability to function, please don't think there's nothing you can do. Grief in itself is not a mental illness, but complex, persistent grief can turn into depression and other mental health difficulties.

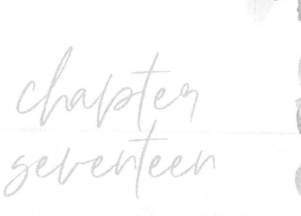

chapter
seventeen

Quick Strategies You Can Use Right Now if You're Overwhelmed

If you learn better with demonstration than from print, and want to see my face, you can access a few of the following exercises via my YouTube channel.

I wanted this chapter to be simple and not too overwhelming, so these are just four of many strategies you could use. If you want more, I have another shorter book, *Birth Trauma Strategies*, which has loads of practical suggestions for coping with birth trauma (or anything really!) using each of your five senses.

If you're a skip-straight-to-the-end type of person, I salute you!

Here's what you need to know about healing, if you've just arrived at this page, or the message throughout the rest of the book hasn't sunk in yet:

1. There's *no quick fix.*

2. Healing is not linear.
3. The treatment of trauma isn't best served by the medical model (in my opinion).

If there was one single strategy I could give you to take all the pain, frustration, shame and guilt away, I'd do it, though arguably neither of us would learn anything or grow. Working on your trauma is kind of like weeding. One approach is to just pull the top off what you can see. That dandelion head that's just poking up through the cracks of your driveway. You're in a hurry, can't be bothered, or just don't want to deal with it right now. So, you pinch off the head and go on your way, knowing full well that you've left the roots behind. Never mind, you'll maybe deal with it the next time.

The other approach is to really get in there. Follow the root down and wriggle that taproot out until you've actually got most of the weed. Here's the thing though. Even if you think you got it all, you expect that maybe there are still some parts you can't see or anticipate. Even if you ripped right through layers and layers of dirt, dandelion seeds may have spread, and dandelions might appear somewhere else unexpected in your garden.

Know that even if you do deep work on yourself, it's unrealistic to apply the approach of 'it's all gone now'. This is why I say the medical model is a poor fit for trauma. Even the most skilled neurosurgeon won't be able to cut your brain open, zap the trauma away and say you're cured. There's no one approach that's going to fix everything.

In saying that, here are some macro strategies you can use right now to soothe yourself:

1. DO SOME SELF-TAPPING USING EFT (EMOTIONAL FREEDOM TECHNIQUE)

Follow my birth trauma tapping videos on YouTube, or come up with your own. If you're limited, you could really just tap into the karate chop point on your hand. Find the fleshy side of your hand underneath your little finger. Hold it as if you're about to karate-chop something. Then, use your other hand to just tap on this point. It doesn't really matter how you do it, the main thing is that you're stimulating this pressure point. Go ahead and tap it while you repeat a self-affirming statement: 'Even though I feel overwhelmed about my birth right now, I choose to love and accept myself'. Keep repeating this, or add in others like 'Even though I feel anxious/angry/scared I'm really proud of myself for working through these feelings'.

You can use tapping in the privacy of your home or in the supermarket queue. The combination of activating an acupressure point with a coping statement builds in a mind–body connection. EFT has become very popular recently. When I first trained in it in 2006 it was considered kind of daggy and 'woo'. The thing I like about it is that it just makes common sense. Acupressure has been around for much longer than most Western approaches to healing. In combination with that, most psychological approaches incorporate some version of positive self-talk, affirmations or coping statements. There is loads of research on the ways in which what you say to yourself impacts your mood, confidence and ability to cope.

I love that it's self-teachable. You don't have to pay an expert to teach you this technique. You can learn it online and then go and teach everyone you know! Tapping is a great thing for kids to watch you doing—monkey see, monkey do! The gift of showing your children how to cope with big feelings in a practical way is a gift that many of us never received as kids, right? You have the power to change that.

2. WRITE A LETTER

I covered this in the last chapter about grief and loss, but I'll repeat it here. The power of writing cannot be denied. A huge part of my own healing has been the opportunity to write down what I know and the tools that I've used so that they may help someone else. Think about what kind of letter you might want to write for catharsis, problem-solving and closure. You don't have to send it or show it to anyone. This is really a chance to say what you need to say without being interrupted and then working towards releasing. You might try:

- A 'fuck you' letter to someone who was in your birth space. A midwife who was rude, an obstetrician who was condescending, someone who wasn't trauma-informed, or who was operating out of fear, exhaustion, scarcity, patriarchy or hunger ... whatever it might be. Get it all out. Swear. Really let them have it. Keep going until you feel some shift. Maybe then you want to read it aloud and burn it. Just don't hang onto it or stuff it in a drawer and forget about it.
- An 'I forgive you' letter. To yourself and/or your baby. For not getting the birth you wanted. For being angry at your body. For not feeling that rush of unconditional love for your baby. For not loving birth. If you've been harsh to yourself and your body, or you've been too afraid to say out loud that you resent your baby, give this one a go. Again, no-one needs to see it. Saying and

writing what you feel doesn't make you a bad parent. It doesn't mean you're ungrateful. As I've said a few times in this book, birth can cause a really complicated trauma response. How many other traumatic events can you think of where people jump in two seconds after you felt you were about to die and remind you that you're supposed to be grateful. Let go of these restrictive boundaries we've placed upon ourselves. You can be resentful of your baby for contributing to your body changing, and still love them.

3. MOVE YOUR BODY: UNHINDERED, UNJUDGED, UNFILTERED

One of the huge things we know about birth and trauma is that a traumatic birth can activate the fight–flight–freeze-appease response. In the wild a mother rabbit who is birthing then suddenly senses a predator will stop birthing and find a safer place and time, if she can. Humans try to overrule our ancient birthing wisdom and primal responses. When the brain senses threat but the body isn't permitted to complete the trauma response (by running away, hiding or fighting), the trauma gets stored rather than released. Being immobilised in birth (through an epidural, caesarean section or even being held down) triggers a trauma response.

When birth memories come up, one of the best things you can do to counter that sense memory of being stuck, trapped and unable to escape is to move. Go for a walk, dance, literally shake it off. Remember your brain doesn't know the difference between what's actually happening and a memory of what's happening. What often happens during memories is that we retreat back into 'trauma time' and our bodies respond as if it's happening all over again, right before our eyes.

Moving the cortisol and adrenaline through your body will help. From a Chinese medicine point of view, moving 'energy' is powerful. Movement helps babies to be born. Movement helps with big emotions. Even if a birthing woman is immobilised (because of a procedure or even just pure exhaustion), having a birth partner or doula just move her legs and massage can help. It's when we stay still and reactivate the immobilisation response that the body and brain get stuck in 'freeze' or defeat mode.

4. USE GROUNDING WITH YOUR EXTEROCEPTORS

One of the most helpful concepts you can learn—not just about trauma, but about yourself—is the difference between exteroception and interoception.

Dual awareness is the ability to see, even if you're upset, having a flashback or feeling distressed, that this is a reaction to something in the past. It's not happening right now. That where you are now is separate from that memory of the past.

Your exteroceptors are the five senses: sight, sound, touch, smell and taste.

The interoceptors are sensations that occur on the inside: balance, heart rate, respiration, if we have butterflies in our tummy, if our muscles ache. This is part of the interoceptive system.

If you are struggling with anxiety or panic right now, you might be seeing reality through your interoceptive senses: for example, my heart is racing and I'm sweating, so I feel unsafe and therefore it must be unsafe for me right now.

Check in to see if you are making an assumption that the environment is unsafe right now without using your exteroceptors as cues. You might feel dizzy and your heart is pounding, but what can you see? The pages of a book? Your laptop or phone? Do you actually *see* anything in the environment right now that is unsafe? Really focus on what you see. A plant? Something out the window? A pile of laundry? See if you can name five things.

Still feel unsafe? That's OK, go to the next sense. What can you hear? What are five things you can hear?

What are five things you can touch? The back of your hand, your shirt? The carpet?

All you are doing here is gently bringing your attention back to the present moment. Instead of telling yourself not to think about the past, all you're going to do is keep grounding yourself in the here and now.

Of course sometimes your intuition might be right, and you're reacting because the environment you're in right now actually is unsafe. But if your life was in danger and you were unsafe right now you might also struggle to really attend to reading a book, so let's focus on situations where you are in fact safe but your brain insists you are not.

You will have used this in the past or might use it in the future, for example if you've ever had a nightmare, or your child or someone in your house has had a nightmare. Often, you'll use grounding— 'I'm here in my bedroom', 'I'm safe'—and you might turn the light on and look around the room. You're reminding your brain where you are.

You can also add to grounding by saying orienting statements. This is a strategy I have used a lot with clients over the years. Simple reaffirming statements like:

'It's 2020 and I'm in my kitchen.'

'It's Tuesday, 2 p.m., and I'm safe.'

As I said, these are just a few simple strategies to get you started. You can search my YouTube and social media accounts for more. As a general rule, deep breathing, using your visual senses to ground yourself, a self-affirming coping statement and doing something physical will help. Nothing is permanent. Although it can feel as though unpleasant feelings and memories will never quieten down, we never maintain the same emotional state.

afterword

If you've made it this far, congratulations. Really. Thank you for taking the time to invest in yourself. It really is the best investment you can make. For me, this book has felt a little like 'Erin Bowe, this is your life'. I've put everything I can think of that might be useful into this book. In the last two and a half years since Lily's birth I've created two birth trauma courses, a podcast, a short e-book, various guest speaking events, one-to-one therapy and coaching work with clients and one-to-one and group mentoring with psychologists. Some of my analogies, exercises and pearls of wisdom are things I have been saying for 15 years. I've often been double-checking that I'm not repeating myself. It's like when you go to see a comedian you like and then they just tell the same jokes you've already heard.

I sometimes worry that people will see the way I talk about my own trauma and think that they can't connect with me. Or that it was easy for me, or that I think everyone should be as poised and professional as I am. There is a line between finding your centre and being calm enough to get your message across on one hand and being completely unapproachable on the other. My business coach is forever telling me to let the wall down and not be so poised all the time. I still have a lot of work to do with dismantling that. I was indoctrinated into a system that said the therapist should never reveal too much about themselves. We are supposed to fade into the background and offer fact and opinion, but not personal experience. I once had a supervisor advise that I shouldn't even wear bright colours or jewellery because it would be distracting and unprofessional. As someone who has always looked younger than I am, I spent a long part of my life trying to get people to take me seriously. I wore black, structured outfits with little or no jewellery. I didn't swear. I'm sure I seemed like I had a massive stick up my arse but I was just trying to find my way. I followed the rules and gave people all sorts of friendly but inauthentic advice about how to cope with kids before I even had any. If that was you, my apologies. Rest assured; karma came back to bite me in the bum for all the 'you just put them back to bed' advice I gave to parents about sleep. My kids are yet to sleep through the night.

In closing, I wanted to reiterate that there are some people who will never 'get' your trauma. It's not your job to convince them. Your goal is to find compassion for yourself. To find strength and growth and realise that you're not broken, and you're not alone. Birth and babies bring out all sorts of opinions. I can't possibly please everyone, and I don't expect people to agree with me all the time. Good art is supposed to challenge us as well as delight us, right? I hope there was at least one phrase that hit you in the guts like a big hug of validation that you needed. I hope there was at least one strategy that you can take to change your life or that of someone else. I hope there was one insight that you have never considered before and are now taking on board to reflect on or research. I hope you will be inspired to take one small step for birth trauma activism. It might be that you stop apologising. It might be that you write a letter to your care provider, hospital or government. It might be that you look for way to use your voice or your actions to elevate the position of people who are the most vulnerable members of our society right now. I hope you share this book and its message with someone else who, right now, at this very moment is being told 'oh well, all that matters is a healthy baby'.

Notes

1   E Bobrow, 'She was pregnant with twins during covid. Why
    did only one survive? Why being Black and giving birth in New
    York during the pandemic is so dangerous', *New York Times*, 6
    August 2020. https://www.nytimes.com/2020/08/06/nyregion/
    childbirth-Covid-Black-
    mothers.html

2   L Gibson, 'Hoosier mothers die in child birth at same rate
    as women in the Gaza Strip: help us find out why', *IndyStar*,
    28 October 2019. https://www.indystar.com/story/news/
    health/2019/10/28/maternal-mortality-indiana-childbirth-
    death-rate/3899877002/
    See also Central Intelligence Agency, 'Country comparison:
    maternal mortality rate', *The World Factbook*. https://www.cia.
    gov/library/publications/the-world-factbook/fields/353rank.
    html

3   See also America's Health Rankings, *2019 Health of Women and
    Children Report: Indiana*, United Health Foundation. https://
    www.americashealthrankings.org/learn/reports/2019-health-of-
    women-and-children-report/state-summaries-indiana

4   S Chapman, 'Indiana has one of the worst rates for childbirth-
    related death', *WTHR*, 20 June 2019. https://www.wthr.com/
    article/news/investigations/13-investigates/indiana-has-one-
    worst-rates-childbirth-related-death/531-c9366a08-be9a-41fe-
    b8ce-18f1d8e37492

5   Australian Institute of Health and Welfare, *Maternal deaths
    in Australia*, 26 November 2019. https://www.aihw.gov.au/
    reports/mothers-babies/maternal-deaths-in-australia/contents/
    maternal-deaths-in-australia

6   UNICEF, *Surviving birth: every 11 seconds, a pregnant woman or newborn dies somewhere around the world*, 19 September 2019. https://www.unicef.org/press-releases/surviving-birth-every-11-seconds-pregnant-woman-or-newborn-dies-somewhere-around

7   Medicare Benefits Schedule Review Taskforce, *Report from the Obstetrics Clinical Committee*, August 2016, p. 20. https://www1.health.gov.au/internet/main/publishing.nsf/Content/24913E0474E75768CA2580180016A033/%24File/MBS-Obstetrics.pdf

8   S Politi, L D'Emidio, P Cignini, M Giorlandino & C Giorlandino, 'Shoulder dystocia: an evidence-based approach', *Journal of Prenatal Medicine*, vol. 4, no. 3, 2010, pp. 35–42.

9   World Health Organization, *WHO recommendations: intrapartum care for a positive childbirth experience*, WHO, Geneva, 2018, pp. 8–9. https://www.ncbi.nlm.nih.gov/books/NBK513812/

10 American Psychiatric Association, *Diagnostic and Statistical Manual of Mental Disorders*, 5th edn, APA, Washington, DC, 2013.

11 National Foundation for Ectodermal Dysplasias, *Learn*. https://www.nfed.org/learn/

12 B van der Kolk, *The body keeps the score*, Penguin, 2015.

13 J Gall Myrick, 'Emotion regulation, procrastination, and watching cat videos online: who watches Internet cats, why, and to what effect?', *Computers in Human Behavior*, vol. 52, 2015, p. 168. doi:10.1016/j.chb.2015.06.001

14 PA Levine, *Waking the tiger: healing trauma: the innate capacity to transform overwhelming experiences*, North Atlantic Books, Berkeley, CA, 1997.

15 DM Wegnerel, 'Ironic processes of mental control', *Psychological Review*, vol. 101, no. 1, 1994, pp. 34–52. doi:10.1037/0033-295X.101.1.34

16 RIM Dunbar (1992). 'Neocortex size as a constraint on group size in primates', *Journal of Human Evolution*, vol. 22, no. 6, 1992, pp. 469–93. doi:10.1016/0047-2484(92)90081-J

17 'Robin Dunbar', *Wikipedia*. https://en.wikipedia.org/wiki/Robin_Dunbar

18 SE Asch, 'Effects of group pressure on the modification and distortion of judgments', in H Guetzkow (ed.), *Groups, leadership and men*, Carnegie Press, Pittsburgh, PA, 1951, pp. 177–90.

19 AS New & B Stanley, 'An opioid deficit in borderline personality disorder: self-cutting, substance abuse, and social dysfunction', *American Journal of Psychiatry*, vol. 167, 2010, pp. 882–5. doi:10.1176/appi.ajp.2010.10040634

20 ES Bowe, 'A comparison of nonsuicidal self-injury in individuals with and without borderline personality disorder', PhD thesis, University of Tasmania, 2012.

21 SJ Francis, RF Walker, D Riad-Fahmy, D Hughes, JF Murphy & OP Gray, 'Assessment of adrenocortical activity in term newborn infants using salivary cortisol determinations', *Journal of Pediatrics*, vol. 111, no. 1, 1987, pp. 129–33. doi:10.1016/s0022-3476(87)80359-1

22 IP Pavlov, *Lectures on conditioned reflexes*, transl. WH Gantt, Allen & Unwin, London, 1928.

23 TS Rotaru & A Rusu, 'A meta-analysis for the efficacy of hypnotherapy in alleviating PTSD symptoms', *International Journal of Clinical and Experimental Hypnosis*, vol. 64, no. 1, 2016, pp. 116–36. doi:10.1080/00207144.2015.1099406

24 N Kar N, 'Cognitive behavioral therapy for the treatment of post-traumatic stress disorder: a review', *Neuropsychiatric Disease and Treatment*, vol. 7, 2011, pp. 167–81. https://doi.org/10.2147/NDT.S10389

25 BN Greenwood, RR Hardeman, L Huang & A Sojourner, 'Physician–patient racial concordance and disparities in birthing mortality for newborns', *Proceedings of the National Academy of Sciences*, vol. 117, no. 35, 2020, pp. 21194–21200. doi:10.1073/pnas.1913405117

26 See note above. For a free-access summary, also see https://www.insider.com/black-babies-more-likely-to-die-when-cared-white-doctors-2020-8.

27 SS Chiarella & D Poulin-Dubois, 'Cry babies and Pollyannas: infants can detect unjustified emotional reactions', *Infancy*, vol. 18, 2013, pp. 81–96. https://onlinelibrary.wiley.com/doi/abs/10.1111/infa.12028

28 SJ Buckley, 'Executive summary of hormonal physiology of childbearing: evidence and implications for women, babies, and maternity care', *Journal of Perinatal Education*, vol. 24, no. 3, 2015, pp. 145–53. doi:10.1891/1058-1243.24.3.145

29 S Buckley, *Hormonal physiology of childbearing: evidence and implications for women, babies, and maternity care*, Childbirth Connection Programs, National Partnership for Women & Families, Washington, DC, 2015. https://www.nationalpartnership.org/our-work/resources/health-care/maternity/hormonal-physiology-of-childbearing.pdf

30 M Odent, 'The fetus ejection reflex', *Birth*, vol. 14, no. 2, 1987, pp. 104–5.

31 M Odent, *The nature of birth and breastfeeding*, Greenwood Publishing, Westport, CT, 1992.

acknowledgements

I would like to thank the beautiful people in my life brought together by synchronicities. When I was pregnant with Stella, I heard that one of my friends from my postgrad program, Sarah Purvey, was teaching hypnobirthing. This led me to meeting Melissa Spilsted. At the first Hypnobirthing Australia conference I attended, I was pregnant with Lily, and was experiencing badly blocked ears, which is one of the weird pregnancy symptoms I get. I barely managed to hear the name of Angela Gallo (now Angel Phoenix) in passing, but my gut said to pay attention. When I looked her up, I instantly knew I wanted her to be my doula and birth photographer. It turns out, I also wanted her to be my business coach, and through her program Heart and Hustle I met some other incredible people in birth work. Through Angel, I met Amberley Harris, who helped me to achieve my goal of becoming confident at breastfeeding. It was also though Angel that I met January Harshe from Birth without Fear. January gave me incredible guidance about book publishing and how on earth to get a book written when you have kids!

At the second Hypnobirthing Australia conference, I was introduced to food guru and priestess Tracey Pattison. I instantly felt like we'd met before. Tracey was a guest speaker at a retreat I ran for pregnant mamas, and her cookie recipe is one I make over and over. When I was finishing this book, Tracey gave me her honest, heartfelt insights from 25 years in the publishing industry, and has never wavered from her encouragement and faith in me to get this book out. Through Tracey, I found Natasha Gilmour and the kind press. Natasha has been everything I'd hoped for (but wasn't really sure existed anymore!) in an editor and publisher. When there is an alignment of values and social justice as it relates to women's voices and birthing a book into the world, magic happens. I'm also so grateful to Dr Juliet Richters for her careful co-editing eye, and ensuring that the feminist and punchy message I wanted to deliver landed clearly.

Thank you to Elle Lynn, who managed to take a handful of disconnected ideas for trauma symbolism and turn it into something beautiful and meaningful. The cover of *More Than a Healthy Baby* is such a far cry from the tokenistic image of a sad-looking woman with a cup of tea looking out of a window.

For my husband, James: thank you for standing beside me year after year (actually, it's coming to decade after decade now!) as I pursue my dreams. There were those one or two years where I actually had a proper full-time job and a salary (remember how miserable I was?), but otherwise you've only ever known me to be studying or pursuing entrepreneurship.

For my mum, Annie Deveney, who always knew I'd write a book some day, and my granny, Susan Gass, who died when I was very small, but who lives on through stories and Scottish catchphrases. One of her sayings was 'whit's fur ye'll no go by ye', which basically means 'what is for you by fate will not pass you by'.

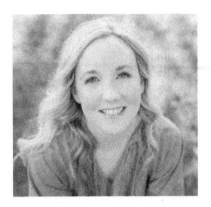

about the author

Dr Erin Bowe is a clinical and perinatal psychologist and coach in Victoria, Australia. Erin had two traumatic births which led her to follow her purpose and passion of encouraging people to find strength and growth after trauma.

She is fervent about empowering women and their families through pregnancy and parenthood through birth debriefing, perinatal counselling, birth trauma training and clinical supervision and is a former provider of Australia's leading childbirth education course with Hypnobirthing Australia.